carbohydrates in Westernized diets portends a future acceleration of these trends. *The Glucose Revolution* challenges traditional doctrines about optimal nutrition and the role of carbohydrates in health and disease. Brand-Miller and colleagues are to be congratulated for an eminently lucid and important book that explains the science behind the glycemic index and provides tools and strategies for modifying diet to incorporate this knowledge. I strongly recommend the book to both health professionals and the general public who could use this state-of-the-art information to improve health and well-being."

—JoAnn E. Manson, M.D., Dr.P.H., Professor of Medicine, Harvard Medical School, and Co-Director of Women's Health, Division of Preventive Medicine, Brigham and Women's Hospital

■

"Here is at last a book explaining the importance of taking into consideration the glycemic index values of foods for overall health, athletic performance, and in reducing the risk of heart disease and diabetes. The book clearly explains that there are different kinds of carbohydrates that work in different ways and why a universal recommendation to 'increase the carbohydrate content of your diet' is plainly simple and scientifically inaccurate. Everyone should put the glycemic index approach into practice."

—Artemis P. Simopoulos, M.D., senior author of *The Omega Diet* and *The Healing Diet* and President, The Center for Genetics, Nutrition and Health, Washington, D.C., on *The Glucose Revolution*

■

"*The Glucose Revolution* is nutrition science for the 21st century. Clearly written, it gives the scientific rationale for why all carbohydrates are not created equal. It is a practical guide for both professionals and patients. The food suggestions and recipes are exciting and tasty."

—Richard N. Podell, M.D., M.P.H., Clinical Professor, Department of Family Medicine, UMDNJ-Robert Wood Johnson Medical School, and co-author of *The G-Index Diet: The Missing Link That Makes Permanent Weight Loss Possible*

"The glycemic index is a useful tool which may have a broad spectrum of applications, from the maintenance of fuel supply during exercise to the control of blood glucose levels in diabetics. Low glycemic index foods may prove to have beneficial health effects for all of us in the long term. *The Glucose Revolution* is a user-friendly, easy-to-read overview of all that you need to know about the glycemic index. This book represents a balanced account of the importance of the glycemic index based on sound scientific evidence."

—JAMES HILL, PH.D., Director, Center for Human Nutrition,
University of Colorado Health Sciences Center

■

"*The New Glucose Revolution* summarizes much of the recent development of dietary glycemic index and load in a highly readable format. The authors are able researchers and respected leaders in the nutrition field. Much that is discussed in this book draws directly from their years of experimental and observational research. The focus on dietary intervention and prevention strategies in everyday eating is an especially laudable feature of this book. I recommend this book most highly as an indispensable source of good nutrition."

—SIMIN LIU, M.D., SC.D., Assistant Professor, Department of
Epidemiology, Harvard School of Public Health

■

"As a coach of elite amateur and professional athletes, I know how critical the glycemic index is to sports performance. *The New Glucose Revolution* provides the serious athlete with the basic tools necessary for getting the training table right."

—JOE FRIEL, coach, author, consultant

Other Glucose Revolution & New Glucose Revolution Titles

The New Glucose Revolution: The Authoritative Guide to the Glycemic Index—the Dietary Solution for Lifelong Health

The Glucose Revolution Life Plan

What Makes My Blood Glucose Go Up... And Down? And 101 Other Frequently Asked Questions about Your Blood Glucose Levels

The New Glucose Revolution Complete Guide to Glycemic Index Values

The New Glucose Revolution Pocket Guide to the Top 100 Low GI Foods

The New Glucose Revolution Pocket Guide to Diabetes

The New Glucose Revolution Pocket Guide to Losing Weight

The New Glucose Revolution Pocket Guide to Peak Performance

■

The Glucose Revolution Pocket Guide to Sugar and Energy

The Glucose Revolution Pocket Guide to the Glycemic Index and Healthy Kids

The Glucose Revolution Pocket Guide to Children with Type 1 Diabetes

■

FORTHCOMING

The New Glucose Revolution Life Plan

The New Glucose Revolution Pocket Guide to Healthy Kids

The New Glucose Revolution Pocket Guide to Childhood Diabetes

The New Glucose Revolution Pocket Guide to Sugar and Energy

The New Glucose Revolution Guide to Managing PCOS

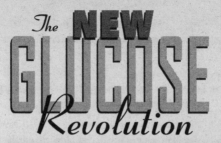

The NEW GLUCOSE Revolution

POCKET GUIDE TO

THE METABOLIC SYNDROME

AND YOUR HEART

Jennie Brand-Miller, Ph.D.
Kaye Foster-Powell, M. Nutr. & Diet.
Anthony Leeds, M.D.

Marlowe & Company
New York

THE NEW GLUCOSE REVOLUTION POCKET GUIDE TO THE METABOLIC
SYNDROME AND YOUR HEART

Copyright © 2004 Jennie Brand-Miller,
Kaye Foster-Powell, and Anthony Leeds

Published by
Marlowe & Company
An Imprint of Avalon Publishing Group Incorporated
245 West 17th Street • 11th Floor
New York, NY 10011

This edition published in somewhat different form in Australia in 2003
under the title *The New Glucose Revolution the Metabolic Syndrome and
Your Heart* by Hodder Headline Australia Pty Limited. This edition is
published by arrangement with Hodder Headline Australia Pty Limited.

The GI logo is a trademark of the University of Sydney in Australia
and other countries. A food product carrying this logo is nutritious and
has been tested for its GI by an accredited laboratory.

Library of Congress Cataloging-in-Publication Data

The new glucose revolution pocket guide to the metabolic syndrome and
your heart/Jennie Brand-Miller...[et al.].
p. cm.
Includes bibliographical references.
ISBN 1-56924-449-9
1. Insulin resistance—Diet therapy—Handbooks, manuals, etc. 2.
Glycemic index—Handbooks, manuals, etc. 3. Coronary heart disease—
Prevention—Handbooks, manuals, etc. I. Brand Miller, Janette, 1952-
RC662.4.N49 2003
616.4'6207–dc21   2003059932

9 8 7 6 5 4 3 2 1

Designed by Pauline Neuwirth, Neuwirth & Associates, Inc.

Printed in the United States of America
Distributed by Publishers Group West

CONTENTS

PREFACE

*U*nderstanding the glycemic index (GI) has made an enormous difference to the diet and lifestyle of many people. Recent studies show that diets rich in slowly digested carbohydrates with low GI values:

- reduce blood-cholesterol levels
- reduce "bad" LDL cholesterol
- increase "good" HDL cholesterol
- reduce CRP (a measure of chronic, low-grade inflammation)
- increase the body's sensitivity to insulin
- improve blood flow
- reduce hunger
- help weight control

In practical terms, this means that:

- our intake of certain foods can influence our risk of heart disease
- a diet rich in quickly digested carbohydrates may increase our risk of a heart attack
- eating more fruit, whole grains, dried peas and beans, and low-fat dairy foods can reduce our risk of heart disease

In this book we will show you how vitally important an understanding of the glycemic index is for your heart health and how easy it is to switch to a low-GI diet. We will:

- explain how the glycemic index is measured
- outline the beneficial aspects of the glycemic index for heart health
- show you how to include more of the right sort of carbohydrate in your diet
- give practical hints to help you make the glycemic index work for you
- provide a week of low-GI menus with nutritional analysis
- list the glycemic index values of more than 400 foods for easy reference

◀ 1 ▶

INTRODUCTION

*H*EART DISEASE IS the single biggest killer of Americans. So big, in fact, that in 2003, more than one million Americans will have a first or recurrent heart attack. And 515,000 of them will die. So what causes this deadly disease? It's often caused by atherosclerosis or "hardening of the arteries." Generally, people develop atherosclerosis gradually, and live much of their lives blissfully unaware of it. If the disease develops fairly slowly it may not cause any problems—even into great old age. But if its development is accelerated by one or more of many processes, the condition may cause trouble much earlier in life.

A CLUSTER OF SYMPTOMS

Heart disease seldom occurs as an isolated condition. For many years the medical profession has been aware that four major illnesses—high triglycerides and low HDL cholesterol, high blood pressure, abdominal obesity and glucose intolerance—often occur together. This cluster of health problems occurs so frequently it has become known in the medical profession as the Metabolic Syndrome or Syndrome X. From a dietary perspective, experts have placed a lot of emphasis on the diet's fat content and how it influences these conditions, since high blood-fat levels are a recognized characteristic of the Metabolic Syndrome. While the type and amount of fat you eat is undoubtedly important to consider (as you'll read about later), newer research suggests that the type of *carbohydrate* plays a significant role, too.

The type of carbohydrate we eat determines the body's blood-glucose response as well as the levels of insulin in our blood for many hours after we eat. We want to avoid the high insulin levels that occur when we eat foods with high glycemic index values. In the long term, higher insulin levels promote high blood fats and high blood pressure and increase heart attack risk.

Because of this, the diet's GI values are significant in the long-term prevention of heart disease and may be equally important to people who already have heart disease.

■

**Eating a lower-fat diet
will result in a higher carbohydrate intake.
What most information on diet and heart disease ignores
is the importance of the
right type of carbohydrate.**

■

◆ 2 ◆

TEST YOUR HEART KNOWLEDGE

*B*EFORE WE GET into the subject of heart disease and the glycemic index in greater detail, take this quick quiz to test your knowledge. Answer true or false to the following questions.

True False
1. ___ ___ All vegetable oils are low in saturated fat.
2. ___ ___ Butter contains more fat than margarine.
3. ___ ___ Americans eat the recommended amount of fat.
4. ___ ___ You should avoid eggs on a low-fat, cholesterol-lowering diet.
5. ___ ___ Moderate consumption of alcohol increases your risk of heart attack.
6. ___ ___ Olive oil is the lowest-fat oil.
7. ___ ___ A cup of milk contains less fat than 2 squares of chocolate.
8. ___ ___ Nuts will raise cholesterol levels.

9. ___ ___ Potatoes and pasta are fattening foods.
10. ___ ___ Cod liver oil will lower cholesterol levels.

The answers to all the preceding questions are false. Here's why:

1. Contrary to popular belief, not all vegetable oils are low in saturated fat. Two primary exceptions are coconut oil and palm or palm kernel oil. Both these oils (which may appear on a food label simply as vegetable oil) are highly saturated. Palm oil is used widely in commercial cakes, biscuits, pastries, and fried foods.

2. Butter and margarine contain similar levels of fat (around 85–90 percent). There is a difference in the types of fats that predominate, however; butter is about 60 percent saturated fat and unsaturated margarine is usually less than 30 percent saturated fat.

3. Americans get about 34 percent of their calories from fat. (The American Heart Association recommends no more than 30 percent of calories from fat for healthy people, and even less for people who have heart disease.) Unfortunately, we're gaining weight, too; most likely because we eat too many calorie-laden low-fat and fat-free snack foods.

4. Eggs are a source of cholesterol but dietary cholesterol tends to raise blood-cholesterol levels only when the rest of the diet is high in fat. One egg contains only about 5 grams of fat, of which only 2 grams is saturated.

5. Moderate amounts of alcohol (about two standard drinks per day) appear to reduce the risk of heart attack. Amounts in excess are harmful to health.

6. There is no such thing as low-fat oil. Oil is 100

percent fat in a liquid form. Olive oil is a suitable choice of oils, since it contains only 15 percent saturated fat. Mediterranean populations, whose major source of fat is olive oil, have low levels of heart disease.

7. One cup (8 ounces) of whole milk contains 8 grams of fat. Compare this to about 4 grams contained in two small squares of chocolate!

8. Nuts have been found to be effective in the prevention of heart disease. While most nuts are high in fat, much of the fat they contain is the "good" unsaturated type.

9. This is a myth that has been around for years. Potatoes and pasta are high-carbohydrate foods, which means they're both good sources of energy for the body. They are rarely stored as body fat.

10. Cod liver oil has not been found to lower cholesterol levels. It is extremely rich in vitamins A and D and should not be taken in large doses because of the danger of vitamin A toxicity.

◀ 3 ▶

THE GLYCEMIC INDEX: SOME BACKGROUND

𝓕OR THE PAST 10,000 years, our ancestors survived on a high-carbohydrate and low-fat diet. They ate their carbohydrates in the form of beans, vegetables, and whole cereal grains, and got their sugars from fibrous fruits and berries. Food preparation was a simple process: They ground food between stones and cooked it over the heat of an open fire. The result? All of their food was digested and absorbed slowly, which raised their blood sugar levels slowly and over a long period of time.

This diet was ideal for their bodies because it provided slow-release energy that helped to delay hunger pangs and provided fuel for working muscles long after the meal was eaten. The slow rise in blood sugar was also kind to the pancreas, the organ that produces insulin.

HOW THE MILLS CHANGED EVERYTHING

As time passed, flours were ground more and more finely and bran was separated completely from the white flour. With the advent of high-speed roller mills in the nineteenth century, it was possible to produce white flour so fine that it resembled talcum powder in appearance and texture. These fine white flours have always been highly prized because they make soft bread and light, airy sponge cakes. As incomes grew, people pushed their peas and beans aside and started eating more meat. As a consequence, the composition of the average diet changed, in that we began to eat more fat; and because the type of carbohydrate in our diet changed, it became more quickly digested and absorbed. Something we didn't expect happened, too: The blood-sugar rise after a meal was higher and more prolonged, stimulating the pancreas to produce more insulin.

HOW THE GLYCEMIC INDEX CAME TO BE

The glycemic index concept was first developed in 1981 by a team of scientists led by Dr. David Jenkins, a professor of nutrition at the University of Toronto, Canada, to help determine which foods were best for people with diabetes. At that time, the diet for people with diabetes was based on a system of carbohydrate exchanges or portions, which was complicated and not very logical. The carbohydrate exchange system assumed that all starchy-foods produce the same effect on blood-sugar levels, even though some earlier studies had already proven this was not correct. Jenkins was one of the first researchers to question this assumption and to investigate how real foods behave in the bodies of real people.

The Pancreas Produces Insulin

THE PANCREAS IS a vital organ near the stomach, and its main job is to produce the hormone insulin. Carbohydrate stimulates the secretion of insulin more than any other component of food. The slow absorption of the carbohydrate in our food means that the pancreas doesn't have to work so hard and needs to produce less insulin. If the pancreas is overstimulated over a long period of time, it may become "exhausted" and type 2 diabetes can develop in genetically susceptible people. Even without diabetes, high insulin levels are undesirable because they increase the risk of heart disease.

Unfortunately, over time, we have begun to eat more "refined" foods and fewer "whole" foods. This new way of eating has brought with it higher blood-sugar levels after a meal and higher insulin responses, as well. Though our bodies do need insulin for carbohydrate metabolism, high levels of the hormone have a profound effect on the development of many diseases. In fact, medical experts now believe that high insulin levels are one of the key factors responsible for heart disease and hypertension. Insulin influences the way we metabolize foods, determining whether we burn fat or carbohydrate to meet our energy needs and ultimately determining whether we store fat in our bodies.

Jenkins's approach attracted a great deal of attention because it was so logical and systematic. He and his colleagues had tested a large number of common foods, and some of their results were surprising. Ice cream, for example, despite its sugar content, had much less effect on blood sugar than some ordinary breads. Over the next 15 years medical researchers and scientists around the world, including the authors of this book, tested the effect of many foods on blood-sugar levels and developed a new concept of classifying carbohydrates based on their glycemic index values.

WHAT IS THE GLYCEMIC INDEX?

The glycemic index of foods is simply a ranking of foods based on their immediate effect on blood-sugar levels. To make a fair comparison, all foods are compared with a reference food such as pure glucose and are tested in equivalent carbohydrate amounts.

Originally, research into the glycemic index of foods was inspired by the desire to identify the best foods for people with diabetes. But scientists are now discovering that GI values have implications for everyone.

Today we know the glycemic index of hundreds of different food items—both generic and name-brand—that have been tested following a standardized testing method. The tables in chapter 21 on pages 113 to 128 give the glycemic index values of a range of common foods, including many tested at the University of Toronto and the University of Sydney.

THE GLYCEMIC INDEX MADE SIMPLE

Carbohydrate foods that break down quickly during digestion have the highest GI values. The blood-glucose, or sugar, response is fast and high. In other words the glucose in the bloodstream increases rapidly. Conversely, carbohydrates that break down slowly, releasing glucose gradually into the bloodstream, have low GI values. An analogy might be the popular fable of the tortoise and the hare. The hare, just like high-GI foods, speeds away full steam ahead but loses the race to the tortoise with his slow and steady pace. Similarly, slow and steady low-GI foods produce a smooth blood-sugar curve without wild fluctuations.

For most people most of the time, the foods with low glycemic index values have advantages over those with high GI values. Figure 1 shows the effect of slow and fast carbohydrate on blood-sugar levels.

The substance that produces the greatest rise in blood-sugar levels is pure glucose itself. All other foods have less effect when fed in equal amounts of carbohydrate. The glycemic index of pure glucose is set at 100, and every other food is ranked on a scale from 0 to 100 according to its actual effect on blood-sugar levels.

The glycemic index value of a food cannot be predicted from its composition or the GI values of related foods. To test the glycemic index, you need real people and real foods. (We describe how the GI value of a food is measured below.) There is no easy, inexpensive substitute test. Scientists always follow standardized methods so that results from one group of people can be directly compared with those of another group.

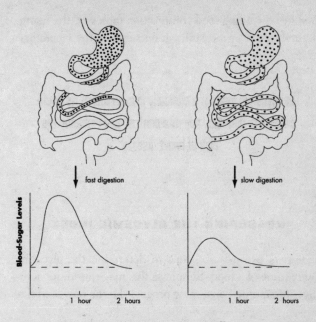

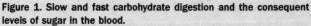

Figure 1. Slow and fast carbohydrate digestion and the consequent levels of sugar in the blood.

In total, 8 to 10 people need to be tested, and the glycemic index value of the food is the average value of the group. We know this average figure is reproducible and that a different group of volunteers will produce a similar result. Results obtained in a group of people with diabetes are comparable to those without diabetes.

The most important point to note is that all foods are tested in equivalent carbohydrate amounts. For example, 100 grams of bread (about 3½ slices of sandwich bread) is tested because it contains 50 grams of carbohydrate. Likewise, 60 grams of jelly beans (containing 50 grams of carbohydrate) is compared with the reference food. We know how much carbohydrate is in a food by consulting food composition tables or the manufacturer's data, or measuring it ourselves in the laboratory.

■

The glycemic index is a clinically proven tool in its applications to diabetes, appetite control, and reducing the risk of heart disease.

■

MEASURING THE GLYCEMIC INDEX

Scientists use just six steps to determine the glycemic index value of a food. Simple as this may sound, it's actually quite a time-consuming process. Here's how it works.

1. An amount of food containing 50 grams of carbohydrate is given to a volunteer to eat. For example, to test boiled spaghetti, the volunteer would be given 200 grams of spaghetti, which supplies 50 grams of carbohydrate (we work this out from food composition tables or by measuring the available carbohydrate)—50 grams of carbohydrate is equivalent to 3 tablespoons of pure glucose powder.

2. Over the next two hours (or three hours if the volunteer has diabetes), we take a sample of their blood every 15 minutes during the first hour and thereafter every 30 minutes. The blood-sugar level of these blood samples is measured in the laboratory and recorded.

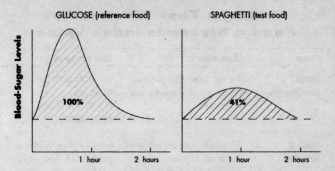

Figure 2. The effect of pure glucose (50 g) and spaghetti (50 g carbohydrate portion) on blood-sugar levels.

3. The blood-sugar level is plotted on a graph and the area under the curve is calculated using a computer program (Figure 2).

4. The volunteer's response to spaghetti (or whatever food is being tested) is compared with his or her blood-sugar response to 50 grams of pure glucose (the reference food).

5. The reference food is tested on two or three separate occasions and an average value is calculated. This is done to reduce the effect of day-to-day variation in blood-sugar responses.

6. The average GI value found in 8 to 10 people is the GI value of that food.

Factors That Influence a Food's Glycemic Index Value

Factor	Mechanism	Food examples
Starch gelatinization	The less gelatinized (swollen) the starch, the slower the rate of digestion.	Low GI: Al dente pasta, brown rice High GI: Overcooked pasta, sticky rice
Physical entrapment	The fibrous coats around beans and seeds and plant cell walls act as physical barriers, slowing down access of digestive enzymes to the starch inside.	Low GI: Pumpernickel and grainy bread, legumes, and barley High GI: Bagels, cornflakes
High amylose to amylopectin ratio*	The more amylose a food contains, the less easily the starch is gelatinized and the slower its rate of digestion.	Low GI: Basmati rice, legumes High GI: Enriched wheat-flour products
Particle size	The smaller the particle size, the easier it is for water and enzymes to penetrate (the surface area is relatively greater).	Low GI: Stone-ground 100% whole-wheat breads and crackers High GI: Enriched wheat-flour products
Viscosity of fiber	Viscous, soluble fibers increase the viscosity of the intestinal contents and this slows down the interaction between the starch and the enzymes. Finely milled whole-wheat and rye flours have *fast* rates of digestion and absorption because the fiber is not very thick or sticky.	Low GI: Rolled oats, beans and lentils, apples, Metamucil® High GI: Rice Krispies, kaiser roll

* Amylose and amylopectin are two different types of starch. Both are found in foods, but the ratio varies.

Factor	Mechanism	Food examples
Sugar	Sugar breaks down into 50% glucose and 50% fructose. Starch, such as enriched wheat flour, breaks down into 100% glucose. Therefore, the presence of some sugar in a food can lower its GI value. Sugar also inhibits the swelling of starch molecules, which also lowers its GI value.	Low GI: Sponge cake, pound cake High GI: Croissant, pancakes
Acidity	Acids in foods slow down stomach emptying, thereby slowing the rate at which the starch can be digested. Examples of commonly used acids are vinegar, lemon juice, lime juice, salad dressings, and brine (used in pickles).	Low GI: Sourdough breads, sourdough English muffins High GI: Enriched-wheat white breads, crackers
Fat	Fat slows down the rate of stomach emptying, thereby slowing the digestion of the starch.	Low GI: Chocolate or white cake from mix High GI: Angel food cake

4

THE PROCESS OF
ATHEROSCLEROSIS

ATHEROSCLEROSIS RESULTS IN reduced blood flow through the blood vessels, which can mean that the heart muscle gets insufficient oxygen to provide the power for pumping blood. That, in turn, can cause angina pectoris (pain in the central chest). Elsewhere in the body, atherosclerosis has a similar blood-flow-reducing effect: in the legs, atherosclerosis can cause muscle pains when you exercise (called intermittent claudication); in the brain it can cause a variety of problems, including strokes.

An even more serious consequence of atherosclerosis occurs when a blood clot forms over the surface of a patch of atherosclerosis on an artery. This process, called *thrombosis*, can completely block an artery, resulting in small heart attacks or even sudden death.

HOW THROMBOSIS OCCURS

The process of thrombosis can occur elsewhere in the arteries, as well; the consequences are determined by the extent of the thrombosis. Whether you develop thrombosis depends in large part on the tendency of the blood to clot versus the blood's natural ability to break down clots. (These two counteracting tendencies are influenced by a number of factors, including some dietary factors, most notably the effect of fatty fish or fish oils in the diet. We'll discuss this in more detail in "10 Tips for a Heart-Healthy, Low-GI Diet" on page 58.)

Those people who suffer from coronary (heart) artery atherosclerosis may slowly develop reduced heart function. For a while the heart may be able to compensate for the problem, so there may be no symptoms, but eventually it will begin to fail. You may experience shortness of breath when you first start to exercise, and sometimes your ankles may swell. Atherosclerosis can also lead to an abnormal heartbeat (palpitations). Remember that your heart isn't the only part of your body that may be affected: you may also notice poor circulation in your legs, which can make your legs and feet feel cold, and exercise may be painful. If your brain doesn't get enough blood due to the poor circulation, you may also be susceptible to a "mini" or even a major stroke.

Modern medicine has many effective drug treatments for heart failure, so this consequence of atherosclerosis doesn't have quite the same serious implications that it did in the past.

WHY DO PEOPLE GET HEART DISEASE?

For most people, atherosclerotic heart disease develops gradually over a number of years. The process begins early in life and is influenced by many factors to which a person is exposed. Over the past few decades doctors and scientists have identified in fine detail the processes that cause heart disease, so they are well aware of most of the factors that contribute to the disease.

Theoretically, atherosclerotic heart disease might be largely prevented if researchers were able to assess everyone's risks during childhood and could encourage them to do all the "right" things throughout the rest of their lives. In practice, though, there's been limited development of ways to screen people early in life for their heart disease risk, and the resources needed to achieve large-scale prevention are just not available.

A great deal is already being done, however, to identify risk factors ("red flags") in healthy people and those with established heart disease. A high cholesterol level is a well-established heart-disease risk factor, as is a low level of HDL—the "good" cholesterol.

More recently, high glucose levels after eating have been shown to be an important but underrecognized predictor of both cardiovascular disease and death from any cause. High levels of glucose in the blood—even temporary increases such as after a meal—have many undesirable effects, because glucose increases the production of free radicals, which are highly reactive, charged molecules that inflict harm on everything close by. For example, free radicals damage proteins, fats, and cellular structures. In particular, they cause inflammation of the cells lining blood vessels. (That's important because we now recognize that atherosclerosis is an inflammatory disease.)

The good news is that you can reduce your risk of heart disease if you take action.

For more information about heart-disease risk factors, see pages 25 to 31.

■

High glucose levels after eating have been shown to be an important predictor of cardiovascular disease. A low-GI diet helps reduce post-meal blood-glucose levels.

■

5

HOW CAN THE GLYCEMIC INDEX HELP?

*T*HE TYPE OF carbohydrate we eat determines our body's blood-glucose response and also determines the levels of insulin in our blood for many hours after eating. Eating high-GI foods raises insulin levels, leading to undesirable health effects, including high blood fat, high blood glucose, high blood pressure and increased risk of heart attack.

Because of this, the GI value of your diet is significant in the long-term prevention of heart disease and may be equally important in the diets of people who already have heart disease. Low-GI diets:

- benefit weight control, helping to satisfy appetite and preventing overeating and excessive body weight.
- help reduce post-meal blood-glucose levels in people with and without diabetes. Keeping blood-glucose levels low improves the elasticity of the

walls of the arteries, making dilation easier and improving blood flow.

◗ can improve both blood fats and clotting factors.

◗ may reduce heart disease risk by increasing "good" HDL cholesterol and reducing the level of blood triglycerides.

◗ reduce total blood cholesterol and low-density (LDL) cholesterol in people with undesirably high levels. Lower levels of total cholesterol and LDL cholesterol are associated with a lower risk of heart disease.

Specifically, studies have shown that HDL cholesterol levels are linked to the glycemic index and glycemic load of the diet. Those of us who tend to eat the lowest-GI diets have the highest and best levels of HDL—the good cholesterol.

HDL cholesterol signals that "bad" LDL cholesterol is being swept away from our arteries, so the higher the HDL levels, the better. Large studies have shown that high HDL cholesterol is the best predictor of a lower risk of heart disease. One of the key features of the metabolic syndrome is a low HDL level.

Furthermore, research studies in people with diabetes have shown that low-GI diets reduce blood triglycerides, a factor strongly linked to the metabolic syndrome. Finally, low-GI diets have been shown to improve insulin sensitivity in people at high risk of heart disease, helping to reduce the rise in blood-glucose and insulin levels after eating normal meals.

By working on several fronts at once, low-GI diets have a distinct advantage over other types of diets or drugs that target only one risk factor at a time.

One study in particular has provided the best evidence in support of the role of the glycemic index in heart disease. The study, conducted by Harvard University, is commonly referred to as "The Nurses Study." It is an ongoing, long-term study of more than 100,000 nurses who provide their personal health and diet information to researchers at Harvard School of Public Health every few years. In this way, diet can be linked with the future development of different diseases. The study found that people who ate more high-GI foods had nearly twice the risk of having a heart attack over a ten-year period of follow-up, compared with those eating low-GI diets. This association was independent of dietary fiber and other known risk factors, such as age and body mass index. In other words, even if the participants ate high amounts of fiber, their risk would still be high if they ate a high-GI diet. It's interesting to note that neither sugar nor total carbohydrate intake showed any association with risk of heart attack. So there was no evidence that lower carbohydrate or sugar intake was helpful.

One of the most important findings of the Nurses Study was that the increased risk associated with high-GI diets was largely seen in those people with a body mass index (BMI) greater than 23. (There was no increased risk for those people whose BMIs were below 23.) But many adults have a BMI greater than 23. The implication? The insulin resistance that comes with increasing weight is an integral part of the disease process. So, if you are very lean and insulin sensitive, high-GI diets won't make you more prone to heart attacks. This might explain why Asian populations, such as the Chinese, who eat high-GI rice as a staple food, don't show increased heart disease risk. Their low BMI and high level of physical activity combine to keep them insulin sensitive and extremely carbohydrate tolerant.

Calculate Your Body Mass Index (BMI)

TO CALCULATE YOUR BMI, divide your weight (in kilograms) by your height (in meters) squared. To simplify the process, go to http://www.cdc.gov/nccdphp/dnpa/bmi/calc-bmi.htm#English) for an online calculator.

PRIMARY AND SECONDARY PREVENTION

When doctors detect the Metabolic Syndrome or heart disease, they have two treatment options available, depending on the state of the disease. First, they treat the effects of the disease (such as medical treatment with drugs and surgical treatment to bypass blocked arteries) and second, they address the risk factors involved to help slow down further progression of the disease.

Treatment of risk factors after the disease has already developed is called "secondary prevention." In people who have not yet developed the disease (those with insulin resistance), treatment of risk factors is called "primary prevention."

Obviously it would be better to give primary preventive treatment in all cases, but luckily, the glycemic index has applications in both cases.

HEALTH CHECKS AND LIFESTYLE ADVICE

More and more people now get regular checks of their blood pressure and blood fats, as well as tests to check for diabetes. All health professionals give patients lifestyle advice to help them stop smoking, exercise more, and eat a good diet. When doctors discover specific risk factors, they give diet and lifestyle advice, but sometimes patients don't follow this advice for very long.

It's especially difficult for patients to follow advice if they aren't likely to feel the ill effects of not following that advice for 10 or more years, and if the changes they need to make are hard to stick to. The person must want to make certain changes and must get support from friends and relatives to keep at it. Also, it's preferable if the person sees the changes in a positive light, thinking to themselves, "I want to do this," instead of "My doctor told me to do this." Any new dimension in heart disease prevention must be seen as a great positive change rather than as a negative one.

HEART-DISEASE RISK FACTORS

*Y*OUR CHANCE OF developing heart disease is increased if you smoke tobacco; have high blood pressure, diabetes or "pre-diabetes" (high glucose levels but not yet high enough to be diabetes), or high blood cholesterol (which may be because you eat too much fat); if you're overweight or obese; or if you don't get enough physical exercise.

SMOKING

Smoking of tobacco is now clearly established as a cause of atherosclerosis; few authorities dispute the evidence. There are, however, some interesting dietary aspects that go along with this risk factor.

Did you know that smokers tend to eat:

- ◗ fewer servings of fruits and vegetables compared with nonsmokers (and consequently fewer protective antioxidants)?
- ◗ more fat and more salt than nonsmokers?

It could be that smokers eat fewer fruits and veggies and more fat because their taste buds have been blunted by smoking and they're seeking stronger flavors. Because these dietary differences may put the smoker at greater risk of heart disease, there is only one piece of advice for anyone who smokes:

■

Please stop smoking!

■

HIGH BLOOD PRESSURE

High blood pressure killed more than 44,619 Americans in 2000. Recent estimates suggest that 25 percent of U.S. adults have high blood pressure, but because hypertension has no symptoms, more than one-third of these people don't even know they have it! High blood pressure (hypertension) is very damaging because it makes your heart work harder and damages your arteries. An artery is not a rigid pipe: it's a muscular tube, which, when healthy, can change its size to control blood flow.

High blood pressure causes changes in the artery walls that make atherosclerosis more likely to develop. Blood clots can then form and the weakened blood vessels can easily rupture and bleed.

Treatments for blood pressure have become more effective over the last 30 years, but it's only now becoming clear which types of treatment for blood pressure are also effective at reducing heart disease risk.

■

Optimal blood pressure (as it relates to heart disease) is less than 120/80.

■

DIABETES AND PRE-DIABETES

Diabetes is, in itself, a further risk factor for heart disease. Diabetes is caused by a lack of insulin—either the body doesn't produce enough, or the body demands more than normal (because it has become insensitive to insulin). Diabetes and pre-diabetes (impaired glucose tolerance) cause inflammation and hardening of the arteries. When glucose levels are raised, even temporarily (such as after eating), oxidizing reactions are accelerated and the level of antioxidants, such as vitamin E and C, decline. In particular, the blood fats are oxidized, making them more damaging to artery walls. The walls become inflamed, thicken, and gradually lose their elasticity. The constriction of the arteries results in increased blood pressure. In addition, high insulin levels increase the tendency for blood clots to form.

The increased risk of heart disease is a major reason why doctors and other health professionals put so much effort into helping diabetic patients achieve blood-sugar control. It's also why all people with diabetes should be checked for the other risk factors of heart disease.

For more information about how the glycemic index can be used to manage diabetes, see *The New Glucose Revolution Pocket Guide to Diabetes*.

HIGH CHOLESTEROL

High blood cholesterol also increases your risk of heart disease. Your blood cholesterol is determined by genetic (inherited) factors—which you can't change—and lifestyle factors—which you *can* change. There are also some relatively rare genetic conditions that can cause particularly high blood-cholesterol levels.

People who have inherited these conditions need a thorough workup by a specialist, followed by lifelong drug treatment. In most people, high blood cholesterol is partly determined by their genes, which have "set" the cholesterol levels slightly high to begin with, plus lifestyle factors, which push the numbers up even more. Body weight also affects blood cholesterol—in some people being overweight has a significant effect on cholesterol levels—so reaching (and maintaining) a reasonable weight can be helpful. The most important dietary factor is fat, and in particular, saturated fat. Some sources of saturated fat include whole milk, cream, cheese, ice cream, butter, red meats, coconut and palm oils, and chocolate.

To lower blood-cholesterol levels, experts recommend low-fat (low-saturated-fat), high-carbohydrate, high-fiber diets. The blood also contains triglycerides, another type of fat that may be linked with increased risk of heart disease in some people. Levels of both cholesterol and triglycerides need to be checked as part of your heart-disease risk assessment.

■

Your blood cholesterol is determined by genetic (inherited) factors—which you cannot change—and lifestyle factors—which you can change.

■

HIGH-CHOLESTEROL FOODS

Many people who aim to lower their risk of heart disease focus on avoiding high-cholesterol foods. Unfortunately, this approach puts the emphasis in the wrong place. Cholesterol itself is concentrated in very few foods (see below) and is not the main cause of our high blood-cholesterol levels. In fact, the amount of cholesterol we obtain from food is generally much less than the amount of cholesterol our body makes on its own. Our body can make all the cholesterol we need, but in certain circumstances, we make more than we need, which causes our blood-cholesterol levels to build up and become a problem.

Those foods that do contain a good deal of cholesterol include:

- Liver and kidney
- Egg yolk
- Caviar

A diet high in saturated fat is one of the contributors to high blood cholesterol. Reducing saturated-fat intake can usually improve cholesterol levels.

LACK OF EXERCISE

Lack of exercise also increases the risk of heart disease. Our cardiovascular fitness improves when we get regular, strenuous exercise (the blood supply to the heart may improve at the same time). Specifically, cardiovascular fitness is improved by *aerobic* exercise, which is activity that makes your heart beat faster so your pulse increases and you breathe more deeply.

Experts believe that we need to accumulate at least 30 minutes each day of this level of exertion to maintain cardiovascular fitness. Exercise is also important in maintaining body weight and has effects on metabolism and some factors related to blood clotting. Clearly, getting regular exercise is important. So don't just think about it, just do it! (For more information about the importance of exercise, see Chapter 9, "Exercise: We Can't Live Without It" on page 41.)

CRP (C-REACTIVE PROTEIN)

CRP in the blood is a new and powerful risk factor for heart disease. It is a measure of chronic low-grade inflammation, indicative of the damaging effect of high glucose levels and other factors on the blood-vessel walls. In women, it predicts future risk of heart disease better than cholesterol levels. Together, CRP and your cholesterol level are a new way for doctors to sort out those at greater risk.

Studies from Harvard have shown that the level of CRP is higher in women ingesting high-GI, high-glycemic-load diets. That's one more good reason to choose low-GI foods!

Normal Ranges For:

Total cholesterol	<200 mg/dL
Triglycerides	<150 mg/dL
HDL cholesterol	>60 mg/dL
Total cholesterol/HDL ratio	< 4.5
Fasting glucose	63–108 mg/dL
Non-fasting glucose	200 mg/dL
Glycated hemoglobin	3.5–6.0%
Insulin	5192 pg/dL

◀ 7 ▶

OBESITY AND
HEART DISEASE

*O*BESITY IS NOW recognized as a serious health concern for a large majority of the American population. In the United States, nearly two-thirds of adults (64.5%) are overweight or obese. Even children are affected by unhealthy-weight concerns: in 2000, approximately 15.3 percent of children (ages 6 to 11) and 15.5 percent of adolescents (ages 12 to 19) were overweight.

Our current obesity statistics result from *chronic* overconsumption of calorie-dense food portions (too many calories in), coupled with *chronic* inactivity (too few calories out). Our genes aren't changing; obesity results from our underactive lifestyle conducted within a food-toxic environment.

We need to tackle the problem on many fronts, including exercise and diet. The glycemic index can play an important role in weight management by helping to control appetite and insulin levels.

WHAT'S YOUR SHAPE?

A commonly used weight-for-height chart called the Body Mass Index (BMI) indicates a range of weights considered healthiest for a particular height, but this reference isn't appropriate for everyone. Athletes, for example, may appear heavy in proportion to their height because of their muscle bulk, but this doesn't mean they are unhealthy. A large mass of body fat, on the other hand, is associated with health risk, especially when the fat is centrally located (waist, tummy, abdomen). Women often carry a lot of fat on their hips, thighs, and buttocks, giving them a pear shape. This fat carries little health risk. You can tell if you have too much fat on your middle by measuring your waist with a tape measure. A waist circumference bigger than 35 inches (females) or 40 inches (males) is too big.

Apple shape   Pear shape

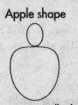   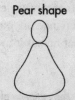

larger waist, smaller hips   smaller waist, larger hips

Figure 3. There is significant health benefit in reducing your waist measurement, particularly if you have an "apple" shape.

■

Are you an apple or a pear?
Your waist circumference should be less than
35" (women) or less than 40" (men).

■

WHY DIETS DON'T WORK

If you are overweight (or consider yourself to be), chances are that you have looked at countless books, brochures, and magazines offering a solution to losing weight. New diets or miracle weight-loss solutions seem to appear weekly. They are clearly good for selling magazines, but for the majority of people who are overweight, "diets" just don't work (if they did, there wouldn't be so many!). At best, a "diet" will reduce your calorie intake. At worst, it will change your body composition for the fatter. The reason? Many diets teach you to reduce your carbohydrate intake to bring about quick weight loss. The weight you lose, however, is mostly water (that was trapped or held with stored carbohydrate) and eventually muscle (as it is broken down to produce glucose). Once you return to your former way of eating, you regain a little bit more fat. With each desperate repetition of a diet, you lose more muscle. Over a course of years, the resultant change in body composition to less muscle and more fat makes it increasingly difficult to lose weight.

■

For the majority of people who are overweight, magazine "miracle diets" don't work. If they did, there wouldn't be so many of them.

■

QUANTITY ISN'T THE ISSUE
—THE GLYCEMIC INDEX IS

Low-GI foods have two very special advantages for people who want to lose weight: they fill you up and keep you satisfied for longer and they help you burn more of your body fat and less of your body muscle.

If you're trying to lose weight, low-GI foods will enable you to increase your food intake without increasing your waistline, control your appetite and choose the right carbohydrates for your lifestyle and your well-being.

THERE'S NO NEED TO FEEL HUNGRY
WHEN YOU'RE LOSING WEIGHT

When you use the glycemic index as the basis for your food choices, you **DON'T** need to overly restrict your food intake, obsessively count calories, or starve yourself. You can lose weight (and reduce your risk of heart disease) *without* feeling hungry!

8

THE GLYCEMIC INDEX AND THE METABOLIC SYNDROME

RESEARCHERS AT THE Centers for Disease Control and Prevention (CDC) estimate that as many as 47 million Americans may exhibit a cluster of medical conditions characterized by insulin resistance and the presence of obesity, abdominal fat, high blood sugar and triglycerides, high blood cholesterol and high blood pressure. Called the Metabolic Syndrome or Syndrome X, the syndrome is a collection of metabolic abnormalities that silently increase your heart attack risk. The list of syndrome features is getting longer and longer, and the number of diseases linked to insulin resistance is growing.

INSULIN RESISTANCE

Insulin resistance means the body is insensitive, or "partially deaf," to insulin: the organs and tissues that ought to respond to even a small rise in insulin remain unresponsive. The body tries harder by secreting more insulin to achieve the same effect, just as you might raise your voice when you talk to a person with hearing loss. So high insulin levels are part and parcel of insulin resistance. Tests on patients with the Metabolic Syndrome show that insulin resistance is very common.

You probably have insulin resistance if you have at least three of the following symptoms:

- high blood pressure
- low HDL cholesterol levels
- increased waist circumference
- impaired fasting glucose
- high triglycerides

Even if you have the Metabolic Syndrome, you may still have total cholesterol levels within the normal range, giving you and your doctor a false impression of your heart health.

You might also be of normal weight (or overweight) but your waist circumference is high (more than 35 inches in women, more than 40 inches in men), indicating excessive fat around the abdomen.

But the red flag is that your blood-glucose and insulin levels remain high after you eat. Insulin resistance is thought to underlie and unite all the features of this cluster of metabolic abnormalities.

You may wonder why insulin resistance is so common. We know that both genes and environment play a role. People of Asian, Indian, or Australian Aboriginal origins appear to be more insulin resistant than those of European extraction, even when they are still young and lean.

But regardless of ethnic background, insulin resistance develops as we age. This has been attributed not to age itself, necessarily, but to the fact that as we get older, we gain excessive fat around our middles, we become less physically active, and we lose some of our muscle mass. It's also likely that diet plays a role: high-fat diets have been associated with insulin resistance, high-carbohydrate diets with improving insulin sensitivity.

Insulin resistance as we age results in the Metabolic Syndrome and gradually lays the foundations of a heart attack and other diseases, including stroke, polycystic ovarian syndrome, fatty liver, acne, and cognitive impairment.

·

WHAT THE RESEARCH SHOWS

Can a low-GI diet help? In a recent study, patients with serious coronary artery disease were given either low-or high-GI diets before surgery for coronary bypass grafts. They were given blood tests before their diets and just before surgery, and during their surgery, doctors removed small pieces of fat tissue for testing.

The tests on the fat showed that the low-GI diets made the tissues of these "insulin-insensitive" patients more sensitive to the hormone—in fact, they were back in the same range as normal control patients after just a few weeks on the low-GI diet!

If people with serious heart disease can improve, would the same happen with younger people? Researchers tried to answer this question when they divided young women in their thirties into two groups: those who did and those who did not have a family history of heart disease. (The women themselves had not yet developed the condition.) After a series of blood tests, the women followed either a low- or high-GI diet for four weeks, after which they had

more blood tests. Then, during surgeries unrelated to
heart disease, doctors removed pieces of fat and tested
them for insulin sensitivity. The young women with a family history of heart disease were insensitive to insulin originally (those without the family history of heart disease
were normal), but after four weeks on the low-GI diet
their insulin sensitivity was normal.

In both studies the diets were designed to ensure,
as much as possible, that all the other variables (total
energy, total carbohydrates) were not different, so that
the change in insulin sensitivity the researchers found
was likely to have been due to the low-GI diet rather
than any other factor.

LOW-GI DIETS IMPROVE RISK FACTORS

Work on these exciting findings continues, but what we
know so far strongly suggests that low-GI diets improve
not only body weight and blood sugar in people with diabetes, but also the body's insulin sensitivity. It will take
many years of further research to show that this simple
dietary change to a low-GI diet will definitely slow the
progress of atherosclerotic heart disease, of course, but
in the meantime it's clear that heart-disease risk factors
improve on a low-GI diet. By the way, low-GI diets are
consistent with the other required dietary changes needed to help prevent heart disease.

■

The message for heart disease prevention:
Eat a low-fat (low-saturated-fat), high-carbohydrate,
high-fiber, low-GI diet!

■

Polycystic Ovarian Syndrome

POLYCYSTIC OVARIAN SYNDROME (PCOS) occurs in women when multiple cysts form on the ovaries during the menstrual cycle and interfere with normal ovulation. Acne and facial hair are part of the problem, as is being overweight, especially around the abdomen. PCOS is often diagnosed when women have irregular periods or find it difficult to get pregnant. It is now known that insulin resistance is often severe in women with PCOS and that any means of improving insulin sensitivity, such as taking drugs or losing weight, will improve outcomes. Some physicians have found that low-GI diets are particularly useful for women with PCOS, but so far, there's little research to back this up. However, since low-GI diets will help reduce weight and have been shown to improve insulin sensitivity in people at risk for coronary heart disease, it makes a lot of sense to try the low-GI approach.

◀ 9 ▶

EXERCISE: WE CAN'T LIVE WITHOUT IT

*D*IET ISN'T THE only way to manage heart disease. Taking good care of yourself requires adopting a few healthy lifestyle habits that need to last a lifetime.

A multitude of changes in our living habits now mean that in both work and recreation, we are more sedentary than ever. Our physical activity levels are now so low that we take in more calories than we burn off, causing us to gain weight and increasing our risk of heart disease. Luckily, exercise is our ticket back to healthy living.

THE BENEFITS OF EXERCISE

Most people could tell you at least one health benefit of exercise (reduces blood pressure, lowers the risk of heart disease, improves circulation, increases stamina, flexibility, and strength), but the most motivating aspect of exercise is feeling so good about yourself for doing it.

Exercise speeds up our metabolic rate. By increasing our caloric expenditure, exercise helps to balance our sometimes excessive caloric intake from food.

More movement makes our muscles better at using fat as a source of fuel. By improving the way insulin works, exercise increases the amount of fat we burn.

A low-GI diet has the same effect. Low-GI foods reduce the amount of insulin we need, which makes fat easier to burn and harder to store. Since it's body fat that you want to get rid of when you lose weight, exercise in combination with a low-GI diet makes a lot of sense!

HOW TO GET MOVING

Getting more exercise doesn't necessarily mean daily aerobics classes and jogging around the block (although this is great if you want to do it). What it does mean is moving more in everyday living. It's the day-to-day things we do—shopping, ironing, chasing kids, walking from the train station—where we spend the bulk of our energy.

Since so much of our environment is designed now to reduce our physical exertion, it's become very important to catch bursts of physical activity wherever we can, to increase our energy output. It may mean using the stairs instead of the elevator, taking a 10-minute walk at lunchtime, trotting on a treadmill while you watch the news or talk on the telephone, walking to the grocery store to get the Sunday paper, hiding the remote control, parking a half mile from work, or taking the dog for a walk each night. Whatever it means, do it. Even housework burns calories!

HOW EXERCISE KEEPS BURNING CALORIES, EVEN WHEN YOU'RE AT REST

The effect of exercise doesn't stop when you do. People who exercise have higher metabolic rates, so their bodies continue to burn more calories every minute, even when they're asleep!

Besides increasing the incidental activity, you will also benefit from some planned aerobic activity, which causes you to breathe more heavily and makes your heart beat faster. Walking, cycling, swimming, and stair climbing are just a few examples. You'll need to accumulate a total of at least 30 minutes of this type of activity five to six days a week.

If you're trying to lose weight, remember that it takes time. Even after you've made changes in your exercise habits, your weight may not be any different on the scale. (This is particularly true for women, whose bodies tend to adapt to increased caloric expenditure.)

Whatever it takes for you to burn more calories, do it. Try to regard movement as an opportunity to improve your physical well-being—not as an inconvenience.

■

Exercise makes our muscles better at using fat as a source of fuel.

■

8 WAYS TO MAKE EXERCISE WORK FOR YOU

Your exercise routine will bring you lots of benefits if
you can:

- enjoy doing it
- feel good about your ability to exercise
- make it a normal part of your day
- keep it inexpensive
- make it accessible
- stay safe while doing it
- do it with someone

HOW DOES YOUR DIET RATE?

To MEET YOUR average daily nutrient requirements, you need to eat a certain amount of different types of foods. If you are trying to reduce your caloric intake, there is still a minimum amount of certain foods that you should be eating each day. These are:

BREADS/CEREALS/GRAIN FOODS— 6 SERVINGS OR MORE

1 serving means:
- 1 bowl breakfast cereal (1 ounce)
- ½ cup cooked pasta or rice
- ½ cup cooked grain such as barley or wheat
- 1 slice bread
- ½ roll or muffin

VEGETABLES—3 SERVINGS

1 serving means:
- 1 medium potato (about 5 ounces)
- ½ cup cooked vegetables such as broccoli or carrot (2 ounces)
- 1 cup raw leafy vegetables, such as lettuce

FRUIT—2-4 SERVINGS

1 serving means:
- 1 medium orange (7 ounces)
- 1 medium apple (5 ounces)
- ½ cup strawberries (4 ounces)

DAIRY FOODS—2 SERVINGS

1 serving means:
- 8 ounces low-fat milk
- 1½ ounces low-fat cheese
- 8 ounces low-fat yogurt

MEAT AND ALTERNATIVES—2 SERVINGS

1 serving means:
- 3 ounces cooked lean beef, veal, lamb, or pork
- 3 ounces lean chicken (cooked, excluding bone)
- 3 ounces fish (cooked, excluding bone)
- 2 eggs
- ½ cup cooked beans

If you prefer larger servings of meat, go ahead—just make sure it's lean. Protein is a very satiating nutrient.

HOW WELL ARE YOU EATING NOW?

Try keeping a detailed food diary for a week. Then, looking at your diet record and using the serving-size guide below, estimate the number of servings of carbohydrate foods you had each day. For example, if you had a banana, two slices of bread and a medium potato, this counts as four servings of carbohydrate.

CARBOHYDRATE FOOD	ONE SERVING IS	HOW MANY DID YOU EAT?
Bread	1 slice	
Low GI:		
100% stone-ground whole wheat, pumpernickel, sourdough, rye		
High GI:		
White, Italian, baguette		
Beverages	about ¾ cup (6 oz.)	
Low GI:		
Apple, tomato, grapefruit juice		
High GI:		
Cranberry juice cocktail, Gatorade		
Cooked breakfast cereals	½ cup cooked cereal	
Low GI:		
Old-fashioned oats, Apple and Cinnamon hot cereal (ConAgra)		
High GI:		
Instant Cream of Wheat, instant oatmeal		

CARBOHYDRATE FOOD	ONE SERVING IS	HOW MANY DID YOU EAT?
Fruit	a handful or 1 medium piece	
Low GI:		
Apples, bananas, oranges, grapes, peaches, strawberries		
High GI:		
Canned fruit cocktail, pineapple, watermelon		
Legumes	½ cup, cooked	
Low GI:		
Lentils, kidney, navy, pinto, lima beans		
Muffins, rolls	½ roll, muffin, or small bagel	
Low GI:		
Apple muffin, chocolate-butterscotch muffin		
High GI:		
English muffin, bagel, doughnut		
Noodles and rice	½ cup, cooked	
Low GI:		
Fettuccine, macaroni, tortellini		
High GI:		
Gnocchi, jasmine rice, arborio (risotto) rice		
Ready-to-eat breakfast cereals	1-ounce bowl	
Low GI:		
All Bran, Complete Bran Flakes		
High GI:		
Cheerios®, Grape-Nuts, Rice Krispies		
Starchy vegetables	½ cup, cooked or 1 cup, raw	
Low GI:		
Sweet potato, squash, peas		
High GI:		
Mashed potato, pumpkin, frozen french fries		
Total:		

Average the number of servings over all the days to come up with a daily average.

Low-GI Eating

LOW-GI EATING means making a move back to the high-carbohydrate foods that are staples in many parts of the world, especially whole grains (barley, oats, dried peas, and beans) in combination with breads, pasta, vegetables, fruits, and certain types of rice.

HOW DID YOUR SERVINGS RATE?

- Fewer than 4 servings a day: Poor.
- Between 4 and 8 servings a day: Fair, but you need to eat a lot more.
- Between 9 and 12 servings a day: Good, could need more if you are hungry.
- Between 13 and 16 servings a day: Great—this should meet the needs of most people.

HOW DID YOUR GI VALUES RATE?

- Fewer than 4 low-GI foods a day: Poor.
- Between 4 and 8 low-GI foods a day: Fair, but you need to eat a lot more low-GI foods.
- Between 9 and 12 low-GI foods a day: Good, but try to add more of these food choices.
- Between 13 and 16 low-GI foods a day: Great—you're eating a low-GI diet.

IS YOUR DIET TOO HIGH IN FAT?

Use this fat counter to tally up how much fat your diet contains. Do a tally for each day and then take an average. Using this fat counter, you will need to compare the serving size listed with your serving size and multiply the grams of fat up or down to match your serving size. For example, if you estimate you might consume 2 cups of regular milk in a day, this supplies you with 16 grams of fat.

FOOD	FAT CONTENT (GRAMS)	HOW MUCH DID YOU EAT?
Dairy Foods		
Milk (8 oz.) 1 cup		
whole	8	
2%	5	
non-fat	0	
Yogurt (8 oz.)		
whole milk	7	
non-fat	0	
Ice cream, 2 scoops (1 cup)		
regular	15	
low-fat	3	
fat-free	0	
Cheese		
American, block cheese, 1 oz. slice	9	
reduced-fat American cheese, 1 oz. slice	7	
low-fat slices (per slice)	3	
cottage, small curd, 2 tablespoons	3	
ricotta, whole milk, 2 tablespoons	2	
Cream, 1 tablespoon		
heavy	6	
light	5	
Sour cream, 1 tablespoon		
regular	3	
light	1	

FOOD	FAT CONTENT (GRAMS)	HOW MUCH DID YOU EAT?
Fats and Oils		
Butter, 1 teaspoon	4	
Oil, any type, 1 tablespoon (½ oz.)	14	
Cooking spray, per spray	0	
Mayonnaise, 1 tablespoon	11	
Salad dressing, 1 tablespoon	6	
Meat		
Beef		
steak, flank, lean only, 3½ oz.	10	
ground beef, extra-lean, 1 cup, 3½ oz., cooked, drained	16	
sausage, frankfurter, grilled, 2 oz.	16	
top sirloin, lean only, 3½ oz.	8	
Lamb		
rib chop, grilled, lean only, 3½ oz.	10	
leg, roasted, lean only, 3½ oz.	7	
loin chop, grilled, lean only, 3½ oz.	8	
Pork		
bacon, 3 strips, pan-fried	9	
ham, 1 slice, leg, lean, 3½ oz.	5	
steak, lean only, 3½ oz.	4	
leg, roasted, lean only, 3½ oz.	9	
loin chop, lean only, 3½ oz.	4	
Chicken		
breast, skinless, 3 oz.	4	
drumstick, skinless, 2 oz.	3	
thigh, skinless, 2 oz.	6	
½ barbecue chicken (including skin)	30	
Fish		
grilled fish, 1 average fillet, 4 oz.	1	
salmon, 3 oz.	3	
fish sticks, frozen, 4 baked	14	
fish fillets, 2, batter-dipped, frozen, oven-baked, 6 oz.		
regular	26	
light	10	

FOOD	FAT CONTENT (GRAMS)	HOW MUCH DID YOU EAT?
Snack Foods		
Chocolate bar, Hershey, 1½ oz.	13	
Potato chips, 1 oz. bag	10	
Corn chips, 1 oz. bag	10	
Peanuts, ½ cup (2½ oz.)	35	
French fries, 25 pieces	20	
Pizza, cheese, 2 slices, medium pizza	22	
Pie, apple, snack size	15	
Popcorn, fat and salt added, 3 cups	9	
Total:		

NOTE: The foods in this list have not been categorized as high or low GI since, with the exception of the snack foods, all other entries contain little or no carbohydrate, and thus are not ranked using the glycemic index.

How Did You Rate?

- **Less than 40 grams:** Excellent. 30 to 40 grams of fat per day is recommended for people trying to lose weight.
- **41 to 60 grams:** Good. A fat intake in this range is recommended for most adult men and women.
- **61 to 80 grams:** Acceptable if you are very active (doing hard physical work or athletic training). It is probably too much if you are trying to lose weight.
- **More than 80 grams:** You're probably eating too much fat, unless you're Superman or Superwoman!

◀ **11** ▶

YOUR LOW-GI FOOD FINDER

A high GI value is 70 or more.
An intermediate GI value is 56 to 69 inclusive.
A low GI value is 55 or less.

	GI VALUE				
	11-20	21-30	31-40	41-50	51-55
11-20					
Peanut Butter	14				
Peanuts	14				
Soybeans	14				
Yogurt	14				
Fructose	19				
Maple Syrup	19				
Rice Bran	19				

	11-20	21-30	31-40	41-50	51-55
		GI VALUE			

	21-30				
Cashews	22				
Cherries	22				
Choice DM™ Beverage, Mead Johnson	23				
Kidney Beans	23				
Barley	25				
Grapefruit	25				
Lentils	26				
Apples, Dried	29				
Prunes, Dried	29				
Black Beans	30				
Hearty Oatmeal Cookies	30				

		31-40			
Apricots, Dried		31			
Butter Beans		31			
Chocolate, Milk, Sugar Free, Fifty50		31			
Soy Milk		31			
Lima Beans		32			
Milk, Skim		32			
Spaghetti, Whole Wheat		32			
Split Peas, Dried		32			
M&M's™ Peanut		33			
Nutella®		33			
Milk, Low-fat Chocolate		34			
Hearty Chocolate Meal Replacement Drink		35			
Ice Cream, Low-fat		37			
Yam		37			
All-Bran®		38			

| | | GI VALUE | | |
11-20	21-30	31-40	41-50	51-55
Cannellini Beans		38		
Navy Beans		38		
Pastina		38		
Peaches, Canned		38		
Pears		38		
Rice, Converted		38		
Tomato Juice		38		
Tomato Soup		38		
Mung Beans		39		
Plums		39		
Ravioli		39		
Apple Juice		40		
Apples		40		
Fettuccine, Egg		40		
Strawberries		40		

	41-50
Bread, Pumpernickel	41
Crème Filled Wafers, Vanilla	41
Black-eyed Peas	42
Chickpeas	42
Peaches	42
Spaghetti, Durum Wheat	42
Chocolate, Milk	43
Custard	43
Pudding	43
Lentil Soup	44
Capellini	45
Pinto Beans	45
Corn	46

	11-20	21-30	31-40	41-50	51-55
GI VALUE ➡					
Grapes				46	
Lactose				46	
Sponge Cake				46	
All-Bran Bran Buds				47	
Macaroni				47	
Baked Beans				48	
Bulgur				48	
Grapefruit Juice				48	
Orange Marmalade				48	
Oranges				48	
Peas, Green				48	
Sweet Potato				48	
Pears, Canned				49	
Muesli				49	
Oat Bran Breakfast Cereal				50	
Rice, Brown				50	
Tortellini, Cheese, Frozen				50	

	51-55
All Bran with Extra Fiber	51
Bread, 100% Whole Grain	51
Mangoes	51
Oatmeal, Old-Fashioned	51
Strawberry Jam	51
Kidney Beans, Canned	52
Linguine, Thick	52
Spaghetti with Meat Sauce	52
Sushi	52
Bread, Sourdough Rye	53
Bread, Stone-ground 100% Whole Wheat	53
Kiwi, Fresh	53

		GI VALUE			
11-20	**21-30**	**31-40**	**41-50**	**51-55**	

	11-20	21-30	31-40	41-50	51-55
Bread, Sourdough Wheat					54
Buckwheat					54
Oatmeal Cookies					54
Pound Cake					54
Rice, Long Grain and Wild					54
Fruit Cocktail					55
Honey					55
Oat Bran, Raw					55
Semolina					55
Social Tea Biscuits					55

◀ 12 ▶

10 TIPS FOR A HEART-HEALTHY, LOW-GI DIET

1. FEAST ON MORE WHOLE GRAINS

Whole cereal grains represent what were the earliest forms of cereal for humans. Eaten boiled or roughly pounded to a flour, mixed with water and roasted, they were a form of slow-release carbohydrate with low glycemic index values, and they were also filling and sustaining. The advent of high-speed roller mills during the Industrial Revolution led to the development of the fine, white flour that we use today. Because the outer seed coat has been removed, the starch in today's flour is readily digested and has a high GI value.

But we can still get the benefit of whole grains in our diet today, with foods such as:

- Barley—such as pearled barley in soup
- Whole wheat or cracked wheat (bulgur)
- Oats and rolled oats for breakfast

- Whole-grain breads (the ones with chewy grains and seeds)
- 100% stone-ground whole-wheat bread
- Whole-grain pumpernickel
- Natural Ovens 100% Whole Grain*

If you're making your own bread, you can add your own GI-lowering ingredients, such as linseed, flaxseed, rolled oats, cornmeal, oat bran, barley meal, cracked wheat, and wheat berries.

*Natural Ovens ordering information appears in the "For More Information" section at the back of this book.

2. USE MORE DRIED BEANS, PEAS, AND LENTILS

Dried peas, beans, and lentils are collectively known as legumes. These are excellent foods that are:

- rich in low-GI carbohydrate
- low in fat
- high in fiber
- low in cost

Because they are high in protein, legumes are an ideal substitute for meat. Introduce them to your family gradually by incorporating them in meals with meat such as in chili con carne, a filling for tacos or burritos, and in soups and salads. You can also try some of the delicious vegetarian dishes made with legumes.

It's easy to use legumes in soups and chili, but have you thought about:

- a mixed three-bean salad
- a can of kidney beans in a spaghetti meat sauce
- hummus dip or spread
- ham and split pea soup

Legume products to look for:

- canned soups with lentils, chickpeas and kidney beans (such as Healthy Choice or Health Valley)
- canned baked beans, kidney beans, butter beans, soybeans
- any variety of dried peas or beans (Goya is a major manufacturer of bean products)

THE SPECIAL BENEFIT OF SOY

Foods based on soybeans also play a beneficial role in our defense against heart disease. There are two components of soybeans with the potential to reduce coronary heart disease risk: soy protein and antioxidant substances called isoflavones.

Soy foods:

- improve our blood fats—lowering the bad (LDL cholesterol and triglyceride) and increasing the good (HDL cholesterol)
- reduce the accumulation of cholesterol in blood vessels by decreasing LDL oxidation

- decrease the tendency to form blood clots or thromboses
- have health-promoting effects on blood vessels

Studies suggest that one to two servings of soy-protein-rich food each day may be sufficient to provide long-term health benefits. Just one cup of soy milk constitutes a serving and can be used as a nutritionally balanced replacement for dairy milk, as long as it's fortified with calcium. Try:

- soy milk on your breakfast cereal
- a soy milk and banana smoothie

3. EAT LOTS OF FRUITS AND VEGETABLES

Plant foods are rich sources of naturally occurring chemicals believed to be involved in disease prevention. Increased consumption of fruits and vegetables is associated with a lower incidence of cancer, cardiovascular disease, and other age-related diseases.

Health experts recommend that you strive to eat at least five servings a day of fruits and vegetables. These foods are an essential source of vitamin C but are also rich in antioxidants and fiber.

Get into a fruit and vegetable habit by:

- including fruits and veggies in all of your main meals
- taking an apple and a banana to work
- preparing one vegetarian meal each week
- making a habit of eating some fruit at home when you relax in the evening

- ordering a side salad with your meal
- preparing a fruit platter for the household to share after the meal
- buying a new vegetable to try each week
- considering fresh, canned, dried, and juiced fruit as sources of fruit for your diet
- chopping fresh pineapple or melon into large chunks and keeping it on hand in the refrigerator
- preparing large amounts of vegetable soups and sauces and freezing in family or individual portions to use later

4. EAT OILY FISH AT LEAST TWICE A WEEK

Oily fish are the best source of long-chain omega-3 fatty acids. These types of fats are scarcely found in other foods and offer valuable benefits in reducing blood clotting and inflammatory reactions. They can help in the prevention and treatment of heart disease, high blood pressure, and rheumatoid arthritis. They are also beneficial in infant brain and eye development.

Fresh fish that are highest in omega-3 fats include:

- Swordfish
- Atlantic salmon
- Silver perch
- Mackerel

Canned fish can also provide substantial amounts of omega-3 fats. Good sources include:

- Mackerel
- Salmon
- Sardines

Smoked salmon is also an excellent source.

■

Aim to eat a type of oily fish at least twice a week as a main meal (just don't fry fresh fish in saturated fat).

■

5. REDUCE SATURATED FATS

Americans eat too much fat in general. Saturated fat, in particular, is believed to be a major cause of high cholesterol levels.

The main sources are:

- whole-milk dairy foods, including cheese and cream
- frozen desserts such as ice cream
- meat, especially processed meats such as sausage, salami, and hot dogs
- high-fat cold cuts, including bologna and liverwurst
- fat spreads, especially butter, cream cheese, and cheese spreads (the exception: natural peanut butter)
- take-out foods, including deep-fried foods, chips, pizza, and pies
- oils such as coconut and palm
- snack foods such as potato chips, chocolate, cookies, and cakes

Make every effort to reduce your intake of saturated fats by eating less of the foods listed previously, and substituting with unsaturated fats whenever possible. For example:

Instead of:	Substitute:
Butter	Monounsaturated spread (canola margarine)
Shortening/lard	Polyunsaturated or monounsaturated oil
Regular milk	1% or skim milk
Fatty meat	Smaller amounts of leaner cuts, such as London broil, flank steak, and center loin pork chops
Regular ice cream	One of the many low-fat varieties on the market
Regular cheese	Low-fat and reduced-fat alternatives

WHAT FAT IS THAT?

The fat in our food is composed of different types of fatty acids. Depending on which fatty acids predominate, we identify the fat as either saturated, monounsaturated, or polyunsaturated. Instead of using the saturated foods listed in the left-hand column below, try one of the monounsaturated or polyunsaturated alternatives listed in the middle and right-hand columns.

Instead of: (Saturated)	Use this . . . (Monounsaturated)	Or this: (Polyunsaturated)
Butter	Canola margarine	Polyunsaturated margarines
	Olive margarine	(such as light tub margarines)
Shortening	Canola oil or margarine	Sunflower oil
	Olive oil or margarine	Safflower oil
	Canola margarine	Soybean oil
	Olive margarine	Light tub margarines

Instead of: (Saturated)	Use this . . . (Monounsaturated)	Or this: (Polyunsaturated)
Palm oil	Peanut oil	Soybean oil
Coconut oil	Avocado oil	Walnut oil
	Peanut oil	Hazelnut oil
Cocoa butter	Canola margarine	Light tub margarines
	Olive margarine	

6. USE LESS SALT

Much of the salt we eat isn't from what we add ourselves: it's from salt already existing in foods. Bread and butter or margarine, for example, contributes much of the salt we eat. Low-salt breads are less than tasty, but low-salt butter and margarines are easy to find on supermarket shelves and aren't noticeably different in taste.

High-sodium foods include:

- canned, bottled, and packet soups
- sauces, meal and gravy bases, bouillon
- ham, bacon, sausages, and other delicatessen meats
- pizza, potpies, fried chicken, and other convenience foods
- pickles, chutneys, olives
- snack foods such as potato chips, pretzels, nachos, popcorn, and salted nuts

7. CONSUME ALCOHOL IN MODERATION

There is no doubt that we all should avoid large quantities of alcohol, but several studies suggest that a moderate alcohol intake can be effective in the prevention of heart disease.

People who drink one or two servings of alcohol per day, but not necessarily every day, show a reduced risk of heart disease, and the effect is greatest among those people with other risk factors for heart disease. This effect may be because alcohol increases the level of "good" HDL cholesterol. Antioxidant substances in red wine that reduce the oxidation of "bad" LDL cholesterol are also thought to be involved.

Please note: three or more drinks per day actually increases the risk of death!

What's a Serving of Alcohol?

Here's how to measure one portion of alcohol:

- beer: 12 ounces
- wine: 5 ounces
- liquor: 1½ ounces

---

8. INCLUDE NUTS IN YOUR DIET

Nuts are a food that many people enjoy but few people eat regularly—a situation that needs to change! Large studies in recent years have found a strong link between higher consumption of nuts and reduced risk of heart disease. Nuts contain a very favorable mix of fatty acids that have a positive effect on blood-fat levels.

Nuts are also a good source of other nutrients thought to protect against heart disease, including vitamin E, folate (also called folic acid), copper, and magnesium.

Because they are so nutrient- and energy-dense, eat nuts only in small quantities. Sitting down to a bowl of nuts may not be such a good idea if you are trying to lose weight, but consuming small amounts of nuts regularly is quite healthy. Try:

- chopped almonds or pecans in granola
- a snack of nuts and dried fruit
- toasted cashews to top off a stir-fry
- a handful of pine nuts or sunflower seeds scattered over a salad

8. USE LOW-FAT DAIRY PRODUCTS

Dairy foods are a great source of calcium, which our bodies need for strong bones and teeth. Luckily, calcium-rich, low-fat flavored milks, puddings, yogurt, ice cream, and mousse make great-tasting snacks and desserts!

Men and premenopausal women should aim to consume 1,000 milligrams (mg) of calcium each day. After menopause, an optimal intake for women is 1,200 mg a day. To get these amounts you'd need to eat at least three to four one-cup servings of a low-fat milk product daily.

One percent and non-fat milk supplies as much (and usually more) calcium as whole milk, so it is entirely suitable for those who want to increase their calcium intake.

- 1 cup of 1% milk contains 300 mg of calcium and only 2½ grams of fat.
- 1 cup of whole milk contains 291 mg of calcium and 8 grams of fat.

■

**Experts recommend whole milk for children
under two years of age.**

■

10. ALLOW YOURSELF A TREAT

We're meant to enjoy our food! So allow yourself to
indulge in a little of whatever strikes your fancy—just
ask yourself first whether it's what you really want.

- your favorite cheese and crackers
- a hot dog at the football game
- bacon and eggs on Sundays
- pizza on Friday night
- a slice of cake at a celebration
- chocolate-chip cookies with a friend

◀ 13 ▶

CHECK THE LABEL
FOR FAT

*U*SE THE NUMBERS on the nutrition information panel to check the fat content of products when you're shopping.

NUTRITION INFORMATION

	per serving	per 100 grams
Energy	121 calories	486 calories
Protein	2.8 g	11.3 g
Fat	6.0 g	24.0 g
Carbohydrate total	14.1 g	56.3 g
Sugars	0.5 g	2.0 g

Across a range of products, aim to buy those with less than 10 grams fat per 100 grams of food. In the example above, the fat content is 24 grams per 100 grams, or 24 percent fat. When the fat content is high, as this is, check the ingredient list for the type of fat:

Ingredients: wheat flour, vegetable oil (palm), tomato powder, salt, skim milk powder, yeast.

The main source of fat in this product is vegetable oil, which is specified as palm oil. From the table on page 65 we can see that palm oil is high in saturated fatty acids, so it would be best to choose another product—with less saturated fat.

Are You Really Choosing Low Fat?

THERE'S A TRICK to food labels that is worth being aware of when shopping for low-fat foods. These food-labeling specifications guidelines were enacted by the United States Department of Agriculture (USDA) in 1994:

Free: Contains a tiny or insignificant amount of fat, cholesterol, sodium, sugar, or calories; less than 0.5 grams (g) of fat per serving.

Low fat: Contains no more than 3 g of fat per serving.

Reduced/Less/Fewer: These diet products must contain 25% less of a nutrient than the regular product.

Light/Lite: These diet products contain ⅓ fewer calories than, or ½ the fat of, the original product.

Lean: Meats with "lean" on the label contain less than 10 g of fat, 4 g of saturated fat, and 95 milligrams (mg) of cholesterol per serving.

Extra lean: These meats have less than 5 g of fat, 2 g of saturated fat, and 95 mg of cholesterol per serving.

WHICH FOODS ARE MOST FATTENING?

Let's compare two everyday foods that are almost "pure" in a nutritional sense.

2 teaspoons of sugar   versus   1 teaspoon of butter

(almost pure carbohydrate)   (almost pure fat)

They contain virtually the same number of calories.

32 calories   versus   34 calories

This means that you can eat three times the volume of sugar as you could butter for the same number of calories! Look at these other examples:

- A small grilled T-bone steak (about the size of a slice of bread) has the same calories as 3 medium potatoes.
- Three slices of bread, thickly buttered, are equivalent to 6 slices of bread with no butter.
- Four Oreos have more calories than a carton of 2% chocolate milk.
- Eating 1 piece of breaded, fried chicken at lunch is the caloric equivalent of 6 slices of bread (without butter).
- For every 1 cup of fried rice you eat, you could eat 2 cups of boiled rice.
- And if you're feeling extra hungry next time you stop for a coffee, consider that 1 glazed doughnut has the calories of 3 slices of lightly buttered raisin toast!

In every case, the highest-fat foods have the highest calorie counts. Because carbohydrate has about half the calories of fat, it is safer to eat more carbohydrate-rich food. What's more, your body is more likely to store fat and burn carbohydrate, so the calories contribute more to your "spread" when they come from fat.

Counting the Calories In Our Nutrients

ALL FOODS CONTAIN calories. Often the caloric content of a food is considered a measure of how fattening it is. Of all the nutrients in food that we consume, carbohydrate yields the fewest calories per gram.

carbohydrate	4 calories per gram
protein	4 calories per gram
alcohol	7 calories per gram
fat	9 calories per gram

◀ 14 ▶

7 DAYS OF HEART-HEALTHY EATING

THIS WEEK OF menus shows you how to achieve a healthy-heart diet with low-GI values. You can use the menus for ideas for your own meal choices or follow them closely to try out the low-GI diet.

Each menu is:

- **low in fat, especially saturated fat.** We've kept the total amount of fat down to provide less than 30 percent of total calories, according to current recommendations. Saturated-fat content is less than 20 grams per day.
- **low in calories.** These menus provide a total daily calorie intake of between 1,400 and 1,700 calories, which is a minimum amount for most people. Let you appetite guide you in terms of quantity.

•

▶ **high in carbohydrate with low-GI values.**
The carbohydrate content of these menus provides
at least 50 percent of total calorie intake. This
means at least 200 g of carbohydrate each day. The
emphasis is on low-GI carbohydrate choices.

Generally, beverages are included only where they make
a significant nutrient or calorie contribution. Supplement
the menus with a range of fluids such as water, tea, coffee, herbal tea, mineral water, and soda with lemon or
lime juice.

We list the recipe ideas for dishes marked with an
asterisk on pages 82 to 84.

MONDAY

GI Value:	48
Total Energy:	1500 cal.
Saturated Fat:	7 g
Carbohydrate:	239 g
Fiber:	40 g

■

Breakfast: One cup All Bran with Extra Fiber™, 1 small banana, 8 ounces 1% milk. Add 1 slice pumpernickel bread toast with 1 tablespoon light margarine (tub margarine) and a cup of tea or coffee.

Lunch: A sandwich made with 2 slices 100% stone-ground whole-wheat bread, 3 ounces tuna, and 1 tablespoon mayonnaise. Finish off with 4 ounces unsweetened canned peaches, and water or decaffeinated diet beverage.

Afernoon Snack: One oatmeal cookie and lemon tea.

Dinner: Two cups minestrone soup (homemade or canned), 2 ounces toasted pita, large mixed salad with fat-free dressing. Water.

Night snack: Four ounces low-fat yogurt and ¾ cup fresh fruit salad.

TUESDAY

GI Value:	45
Total Energy:	1500 cal.
Saturated Fat:	12 g
Carbohydrate:	228 g
Fiber:	19 g

■

Breakfast: Two slices 100% stone-ground whole-wheat toast with 4 tablespoons light ricotta cheese. Finish off with 1 small pear and 1 cup of hot chocolate made with 1% milk.

Lunch: Try a sandwich made with 2 slices pumpernickel bread, 1 ounce boiled ham and 1 ounce reduced-fat cheddar cheese and 2 crispy pickle spears on the side. Finish with ¾ cup fresh fruit salad and water or decaffeinated diet beverage.

Afternoon snack: One small low-fat apple-cinnamon muffin.

Dinner: Four ounces Barbecued Beef Kebabs* with ¾ cup Quick Rice Combo**. Finish with large tossed salad with fat-free dressing and beverage.

Night snack: One-half cup low-fat ice cream.

*See recipe on page 84.
** See recipe on page 83.

WEDNESDAY

GI Value:	43
Total Energy:	1450 cal.
Saturated Fat:	10 g
Carbohydrate:	218 g
Fiber:	29 g

■

Breakfast: One cup old-fashioned oatmeal made with 8 ounces 1% milk. Add ½ grapefruit; tea or coffee.

Lunch: Two slices 100% stone-ground whole-wheat bread spread with 2 tablespoons natural peanut butter and 1 tablespoon all-fruit jelly. Finish with 1 cup grapes and water or decaffeinated diet beverage.

Afternoon snack: Eight ounces fat-free fruited yogurt.

Dinner: Vegetarian Chili Fajita* and large tossed salad with fat-free dressing and water.

Night snack: One ounce dry-roasted almonds and 1 cup of tea.

*See recipe on page 83.

THURSDAY

GI Value:	46
Total Energy:	1600 cal.
Saturated Fat:	9 g
Carbohydrate:	207g
Fiber:	42 g

■

Breakfast: Toast 2 slices 100% stoneground whole-wheat bread and top with 1 tablespoon of light (tub) margarine. Add 1 soft-boiled egg, 1 medium peach, and cup of tea or coffee.

Lunch: Two cups lentil soup (commercial or home-made) with tossed salad made with 2 tablespoons vinaigrette. Finish off with water or tea.

Afternoon snack: An orange.

Dinner: One Salmon Cake* served with 1 cup frozen vegetable medley, 1 cup rice pilaf, and beverage.

Night snack: One-half cup fat-free chocolate pudding.

*See recipe on page 83.

FRIDAY

GI Value:	41
Total Energy:	1400 cal.
Saturated Fat:	11 g
Carbohydrate:	226 g
Fiber:	15 g

■

Breakfast: One cup Special K™ with 8 ounces 1% milk and ½ banana. Tea or coffee.

Lunch: Sandwich made with 2 slices sourdough rye bread, 2 ounces smoked salmon and 1 tablespoon light cream cheese. Add 1 cup tomato, cucumber, and onion salad with 2 tablespoons reduced-fat Italian dressing and water to drink.

Afternoon snack: One oatmeal cookie and 6 ounces non-fat fruited yogurt.

Dinner: One-and-a-half cups Easy Creamy Pasta* with tomato sauce, ½ cup green beans and 1 small baked apple with cinnamon for dessert. Top off with water or decaffeinated diet beverage.

Night snack: One-half cup low-fat frozen yogurt (soft serve).

*See recipe on page 82.

SATURDAY

GI Value:	45
Total Energy:	1650 cal.
Saturated Fat:	15 g
Carbohydrate:	236 g
Fiber:	27g

■

Breakfast: Three 4-inch buckwheat pancakes, 1 table-spoon strawberry jam, 2 strips bacon, and one small apple. Coffee or tea.

Lunch: Inside a 2-ounce tortilla, wrap 1 cup raw spinach, ½ cup diced tomato, 2 ounces turkey, 1 ounce cheese and 2 tablespoons light mayonnaise. Finish off with a large pear and water.

Afternoon snack: One medium apple.

Dinner: Four ounces London broil, 1 medium sweet potato, 1 cup steamed broccoli with 1 teaspoon light (tub) margarine and a beverage.

Night snack: Eight ounces apple juice with 3 Social Tea biscuits.

SUNDAY

GI Value:	46
Total Energy:	1600 cal.
Saturated Fat:	13 g
Carbohydrate:	181 g
Fiber:	21 g

■

Breakfast: Three-quarters cup fresh fruit salad, 4 ounces low-fat fruited yogurt, 2 ounces apple-cinnamon muffin. Tea or coffee.

Lunch: Two slices pumpernickel bread, a 2-egg omelet with diced tomatoes and shallots, and 2 tablespoons shredded cheddar cheese. Add a tossed green salad with fat-free dressing and beverage.

Afternoon snack: One banana.

Dinner: Broil a 6-ounce fish fillet (such as sole, flounder, orange roughy, or catfish) drizzled with one tablespoon olive oil, lemon juice, salt, and pepper. Serve with 6 ounces canned new potatoes and 1 cup (12 spears) asparagus or other seasonal vegetables. Top off with cup of lemon tea.

Night snack: Two ounces trail mix.

◀ 15 ▶

QUICK MEAL IDEAS

*T*HESE RECIPE IDEAS are used in the previous menu plans. The quantities of each ingredient are only a rough guide and can easily be adjusted to taste.

EASY CREAMY PASTA

Cook 8 ounces broad fettuccine noodles according to box instructions. Combine ¼ cup of part-skim ricotta, ¼ cup of non-fat plain yogurt, ¼ cup of grated Parmesan and 1 tablespoon of margarine. Stir this mixture through the drained pasta, adding some sautéed onion and garlic for extra flavor if desired. A quick topping idea: commercial pasta sauce.

SERVES 4.

■

VEGETARIAN CHILI FAJITA

Sauté a diced onion, a clove of crushed garlic, and thin strips of green pepper. Add 4 thinly sliced mushrooms and oregano to taste and cook 5 minutes. Stir in a small can of red kidney beans. Sprinkle a 2-ounce tortilla with ½ cup of shredded reduced-fat cheddar or Monterey jack cheese. Spoon the bean mixture onto the tortilla and fold it over to enclose the ingredients. Pour about ½ cup of salsa or picante sauce over tortilla and top with another ½ cup of cheese. Bake 10–15 minutes in hot oven.

SERVES 4.

SALMON CAKES

Combine a 6-ounce can of salmon with ½ onion (finely diced), ½ cup mashed potato, 2 teaspoons chopped parsley, and 1 egg. Shape into patties and fry in a pan sprayed with cooking spray.

SERVES 2.

QUICK RICE COMBO

Fry 2 strips of trimmed diced bacon, 1 diced small red pepper, 2 chopped shallots, and 1 cup of frozen peas. Add 2 cups of cooked Uncle Ben's Converted rice, drizzle with soy sauce, and serve.

SERVES 4.

BARBECUED BEEF KEBABS

Marinate approximately 1 pound of cubed beef (e.g., top round or sirloin) in ½ cup red wine, 1 tablespoon vinegar, 1 tablespoon olive oil, 1 teaspoon Worcestershire sauce, 2 tablespoons ketchup, crushed garlic, and black pepper. Thread the meat cubes onto the skewer alternately with mushrooms and pepper and onion strips. Grill or barbecue and serve with Quick Rice Combo.

SERVES 4.

∎

◀ 16 ▶

A GI SUCCESS STORY

To HELP ILLUSTRATE how a low-GI diet can improve your heart-disease risk factors, dietitian Johanna Burani, M.S., R.D., C.D.E., offers this real-life example from her own practice. Many of Johanna's patients have lost weight, controlled their diabetes, and gained overall better health by choosing a low-GI way of life.

CASE STUDY:
"Jay"

Age:	66
Height:	5'10
Weight:	171 pounds

(healthy weight range for his height)

BACKGROUND

Jay is a retired letter carrier who used to smoke and drink until he quit some twenty years ago. He hates to exercise. Jay suffers from type 2 diabetes and has elevated blood fats. He has already undergone successful triple bypass surgery.

Jay's typical diet before surgery:

Breakfast: Fried eggs, Taylor ham, home fries, and several cups of coffee (with half-and-half and sugar) and buttered toast

Lunch: A salami sandwich on a hard roll, donut, and Coke

Snack: Several pieces of coffee cake with coffee

Dinner: Steak, baked potato with butter, salad, apple pie a la mode, Coke

Late-night snack: Three or four scoops of ice cream (large bowl)

Jay's "Before" Nutritional Analysis:	
Calories:	4250
Carbohydrate:	447 g (42%)
Protein:	265 g (25%)
Fat:	156 g (33%)
GI Value:	72

Johanna's nutritional assessment:

To maximize the health benefits of his successful heart surgery, it was paramount for Jay to decrease his total caloric intake, take a serious look at his dietary sources of fat (specifically saturated fat), and find ways to incorporate a minimum of five servings of fruits and vegetables into his diet every day.

GI-specific counseling:

Jay's carbohydrate intake (nearly 1800 calories) came almost exclusively from refined starches (such as white bread, rolls, baked goods, and sugar). The rapid digestion of these foods kept Jay hungry, so he ate large meals and snacks. He didn't think there was any problem with this way of eating since he wasn't overweight. The more calories he consumed, however, the greater his cholesterol and saturated fat intake was, which eventually clogged three of his arteries, necessitating bypass surgery.

Solution: The low-GI, high-fiber foods that he would incorporate into his diet would enable Jay to feel full longer—as the higher-fat foods did previously—but without the negative impact on the health of his once-compromised heart. A low-GI diet would have the added benefit of improving Jay's diabetes control.

Jay's new, low-GI menu:

Johanna put Jay on a 2,800-calorie-a-day, low-GI meal plan for a 4-week transitional period, after which Jay followed a 2,000-calorie-a-day menu eating meals such as these:

Breakfast: Two slices sourdough rye toast with 1 tablespoon light (tub) margarine, Egg Beater omelet with mushrooms and onions, small glass of grapefruit juice, reduced-caffeine coffee with Equal and fat-free half-and-half

Snack: Eight-ounce glass 1% milk (with 2 ounces cold coffee), 2 or 3 graham crackers

Lunch: A double-decker sandwich (3 slices sourdough rye bread, 2 slices boiled ham, 2 slices reduced-fat cheese, large sliced cucumber), fat-free, no-sugar-added cooked butterscotch pudding, seltzer

Snack: Diet Coke (caffeine-free)

Dinner: One cup rice pilaf, 6 ounces broiled scallops in wine and lemon sauce, 1 cup cooked wax beans, a handful of grapes, seltzer

Snack: Low-fat apple-cinnamon muffin, herbal tea

Jay's "After" Nutritional Analysis:

Calories:	2000
Carbohydrate:	287 g (56%)
Protein:	110 g (24%)
Fat:	50 g (24%)
GI value:	52

Jay's winning results:

It's been more than seven years since Jay's bypass surgery. He continues to follow the low-fat, high-fiber, low-GI guidelines that Johanna gave him after his surgery. He's also maintained a healthy weight, which is currently 172½ pounds. His blood pressure remains good without medication and his blood sugars have been excellent long enough for his doctor to suggest that he try cutting back from two pills a day to just one. He successfully completed his cardiac rehabilitation program and needs to visit his cardiologist only once a year.

Jay's comments:

"I feel great; nothing bothers me. I hate to exercise, but my wife hollers at me if I don't, so I take a short walk every day."

◀ 17 ▶

YOUR QUESTIONS ANSWERED

I have heart disease and my doctor has told me to lose weight. How can a high-carbohydrate–low-GI diet help me shed pounds?

Because low-GI diets lower insulin levels, over the long term you'll burn more—and store less—fat. (Insulin determines how much fat we store and burn.) And . . .

- ▶ You're less likely to overeat low-GI carbohydrates, because they're bulky and filling. Consider them natural appetite suppressants!
- ▶ A low-GI diet offers you plenty of food choices, so you're less likely to feel deprived. Unlike diets that restrict certain foods, a low-GI diet is easy to live with.

Can I still lose weight eating as much carbohydrate as I want?

Possibly not. We recommend a high carbohydrate intake and a low fat intake. While carbohydrate is not usually stored as fat, if you are eating more total energy than your body requires, then the carbohydrate will be used as a source of fuel in preference to fat. This would have the effect of limiting the breakdown of body fat stores. The idea is to eat enough energy in total to satisfy your appetite (eating low-GI foods helps) and nutritional requirements, but not more than you need. An increase in your activity level will help burn up body fat as it is used as an additional fuel.

I've always heard that sugar is fattening. Is it?

No. Sugar has no special fattening properties—in fact, it is no more likely to be turned into fat than any other carbohydrate. Sugar, which you'll often find in foods high in calories and fat, may sometimes seem to be "turned into fat," but it's the total number of calories you're consuming rather than the sugar in those calorie-dense foods that may contribute to new stores of fat.

Why are diets that disregard widely accepted nutritional guidelines so fashionable right now?

Several best-selling books have been published promoting high-protein diets and generating a lot of publicity. They have been seized upon as a viable weight, loss panacea. But the fact is: diets that limit major food groups do not work over the long haul.

What are the side effects of a high-protein diet?

The body cannot process large quantities of protein, so excess waste is produced that can overburden the kidneys. Not only can some high-protein diets make existing kidney problems worse, but they also can cause mild renal failure to progress faster. Some high-protein diets are also harmful for elderly people and anyone with high blood pressure or diabetes. High-protein, high-fat diets can lead to high cholesterol, and heart disease, and increase the risk of heart attack. Further, some high-protein diets reduce the intake of important vitamins, minerals, fiber, and trace elements. They also lack fiber, which may lead to constipation.

Overweight people with heart disease need to shed pounds. Why do people on high-protein diets lose weight?

Because they make people lose water weight. Overweight people need to lose body fat—not muscle or water. And the way to do this is to eat a balanced diet of low-GI carbohydrates and burn more calories than we take in.

◀ 18 ▶

THE LOW-GI CHECKLIST

*G*OING GROCERY SHOPPING? Bring this list with you. It will help you choose low- and intermediate-GI foods quickly and easily.

BREADS

100% stone-ground whole-wheat
100% Whole Grain, Natural Ovens (see page 130 for ordering information)
Flatbread, Indian
Happiness, Natural Ovens
Hearty 7 Grain
Hunger Filler, Natural Ovens
Muesli, made from mix
Natural Wheat, Natural Ovens
Pita, whole-wheat
Pumpernickel, whole-grain
Rye

Sourdough
Sourdough rye
Soy & Linseed, machine mix
Spelt, multigrain

BREAKFAST CEREALS

All-Bran with Extra Fiber™
Bran Buds with Psyllium™
Bran Buds™, Kellogg's
Bran Chex™, Kellogg's
Bran Flakes™, Complete®, Kellogg's
Cereal, hot, apple and cinnamon, ConAgra
Cream of Wheat™, regular, Nabisco
Frosted Flakes™, Kellogg's
Froot Loops™, Kellogg's
Just Right™, Kellogg's
Life™, Quaker Oats
Muesli, natural
Muesli, toasted
Nutrigrain™, Kellogg's
Oat bran
Oat bran, raw
Oatmeal, old-fashioned, cooked
Puffed Wheat, Quaker Oats
Raisin Bran™, Kellogg's
Rice bran
Special K™, Kellogg's

COOKIES AND CAKES

Biscuits, Social Tea™
Bread, banana

Cake, chocolate, with chocolate frosting
Cake, pound
Cake, sponge
Cake, vanilla
Cookies, Arrowroot
Cookies, Hearty Oatmeal, FIFTY50
Cookies, oatmeal
Cookies, Oatmeal, Sugar Free, FIFTY50
Cookies, shortbread
Muffin, apple cinnamon, from mix*
Wafers, vanilla, creme filled, FIFTY50

DAIRY PRODUCTS AND ALTERNATIVES

Custard, homemade
Ice cream, regular
Milk, low-fat, chocolate, with aspartame
Milk, low-fat, chocolate, with sugar
Milk, skim
Milk, whole
Mousse, butterscotch, low-fat, Nestlé
Mousse, chocolate, low-fat, Nestlé
Mousse, French vanilla, low-fat, Nestlé
Mousse, hazelnut, low-fat, Nestlé
Mousse, mango, low-fat, Nestlé
Mousse, mixed berry, low-fat, Nestlé
Mousse, strawberry, low-fat, Nestlé
Pudding, instant, chocolate, made with milk
Pudding, instant, vanilla, made with milk
Soy milk, reduced-fat
Soy milk, whole
Yogurt, low-fat, fruit, with aspartame

*Foods containing fat in excess of American Heart Association guidelines. Use these only once in a while and in small amounts.

Yogurt, low-fat, fruit, with sugar
Yogurt, non-fat, French vanilla, with sugar
Yogurt, non-fat, strawberry, with sugar

FRUIT AND FRUIT PRODUCTS

Apple, fresh
Apricot, fresh
Banana, fresh
Cantaloupe, fresh
Cherries, fresh
Figs, dried
Fruit cocktail, canned
Grapefruit, fresh
Grapes, fresh
Kiwi, fresh
Mango, fresh
Orange, fresh
Papaya, fresh
Peach, canned in natural juice
Peach, fresh
Pear, canned in pear juice
Pineapple, fresh
Pear, fresh
Plum, fresh
Prunes, pitted
Raisins/sultanas
Strawberries, fresh
Strawberry jam

GRAINS

Barley, cracked
Barley, pearled

Barley, rolled
Buckwheat
Buckwheat groats
Bulgur
Corn, canned, no salt added
Corn, fresh
Couscous
Rice, arborio (risotto)
Rice, Basmati
Rice, brown
Rice, Cajun Style, Uncle Ben's®
Rice, Garden Style, Uncle Ben's®
Rice, Long Grain and Wild, Uncle Ben's®
Rice, parboiled, Converted, white, cooked 20–30 minutes, Uncle Ben's®
Rice, parboiled, Long Grain, cooked 10 minutes, Uncle Ben's®

JUICES

Apple, with sugar or artificial sweetener
Carrot, fresh
Grapefruit, unsweetened
Pineapple, unsweetened
Tomato, canned, no added sugar

LEGUMES

Beans, baked, canned
Beans, butter, dried and cooked
Beans, kidney, canned
Beans, lima, baby, frozen
Beans, mung, cooked

Beans, navy, dried and cooked
Beans, pinto, cooked
Beans, soy, canned
Chickpeas/garbanzo beans, canned
Lentils, green, dried and cooked
Lentils, red, dried and cooked
Peas, black-eyed
Peas, split, yellow, cooked

> Note: Canned legumes have higher GI values than the boiled varieties because the temperatures and pressures used in the canning process increase the digestibility of the starch. But, canned legumes are still an excellent low-fat, high-fiber, nutrient-rich, low-GI choice!

NOODLES AND PASTA

Capellini
Fettuccine, egg
Gluten-free noodles, cornstarch
Instant noodles
Linguine, thick, fresh, durum wheat, white
Linguine, thin, fresh, durum wheat
Macaroni, plain, cooked
Mung bean, Lungkow beanthread
Ravioli
Rice, dried, cooked
Rice, fresh, cooked
Spaghetti, cooked 5 minutes
Spaghetti, cooked 10 minutes, Barilla
Spaghetti, cooked 22 minutes
Spaghetti, protein-enriched, cooked 7 minutes
Spaghetti, whole wheat
Spirali, cooked, durum wheat

Star pastina, cooked 5 minutes
Tortellini
Udon, plain, reheated 5 minutes
Vermicelli

SNACK FOODS

Apple cinnamon snack bar, ConAgra
Cashews
Chocolate bar, milk, Cadbury's
Chocolate bar, milk, Dove®, Mars
Chocolate bar, milk, Nestlé
Chocolate bar, white, Milky Bar®
Chocolate bar, Snickers®
Corn chips, plain, salted, Doritos™
M&M's®, peanut
Nougat
Nutella®, chocolate hazelnut spread
Peanut butter & chocolate-chip snack bar
Peanuts
Pecans
Potato chips, plain, salted
Twix® Cookie Bar, caramel

SOUPS

Black bean, canned
Green pea, canned
Lentil, canned
Minestrone, canned, ready-to-serve
Tomato, canned

STARCHY VEGETABLES

Corn, canned, no salt added
Peas, frozen, cooked
Potato, new, canned
Potato, sweet
Yam

VEGETABLES

Artichoke
Avocado
Beet
Bok choy
Broccoli
Cabbage
Carrots, peeled, cooked
Cassava (yucca), cooked with salt
Cauliflower
Celery
Corn, canned, no salt added
Corn, sweet, cooked
Cucumber
French beans (runner beans)
Leafy greens
Lettuce
Peas, frozen, cooked
Pepper
Potato, boiled/canned
Potato, new, canned
Squash
Taro
Yam

◀ 19 ▶

CUTTING THE FAT: YOUR A TO Z GUIDE

*A*S WE HAVE said constantly throughout this book, it is important to eat a high-carbohydrate and low-fat diet. The following practical tips, which we have set out in an easy A to Z format, will help you reduce the fat content of some of your favorite recipes while lowering their GI value.

Alcohol

Although excessive alcohol consumption can be fattening, as an ingredient in a recipe, alcohol itself won't create a high-calorie dish. Alcohol evaporates during cooking, so you lose the calories and are left with the flavor. A little wine in a sauce can give a delicious flavor, and sherry in an Asian-style marinade is essential.

Bacon

Bacon is a valuable ingredient in many dishes because of the flavor it offers. You can make a little bacon go a long way by trimming off all fat and chopping it finely. Lean ham is often a more economical and leaner way to go. In casseroles and soups, a ham bone imparts a fine flavor without much fat.

Cheese

Several commonly used cheeses, such as American, cheddar, and blue, contain more than 70 percent of their calories as fat. Although there are a number of fat-reduced cheeses available, many of these lose a lot in flavor for a small reduction in fat. It is worth comparing fat per ounce between brands to find the tastiest one with the lowest fat content. Alternatively, a sprinkle of a very tasty grated cheese or Parmesan may do the job.

Part-skim ricotta and cottage cheeses are lower-fat alternatives to butter on a sandwich. It's worth trying some fresh part-skim ricotta from a deli—you may find the texture and flavor more acceptable than that of the ricotta available in containers in the supermarket. Flavored cottage cheeses are ideal low-fat toppings for crackers. Try ricotta in lasagna instead of a creamy white sauce.

Cream and sour cream

Keep to very small amounts, as these are high in saturated fat. Substitute non-fat sour cream, which tastes very similar to the full-fat variety. A 16-ounce container of heavy cream can be poured into ice-cube trays and frozen, providing small servings of cream easily when you need it. Adding one ice-cube block (1 oz.) of cream to a dish adds only 5½ grams of fat.

Dried beans, peas, and lentils

These are all low in fat and very nutritious. Incorporating them in a recipe, perhaps as a partial substitution for meat, will lower the fat content of the finished product. Canned beans, chickpeas, and lentils are now widely available. They are very convenient to use and a great time saver. They are comparable in food value to the dried ones that you soak and cook yourself.

Eggs

Be conscious of eggs in a recipe, as they can add fat. Sometimes just the beaten egg white can be substituted for the whole egg, or use real egg substitute.

Filo pastry

Unlike most other pastry, filo (also known as phyllo) is low in fat. To keep it that way, brush between the sheets with skim milk instead of melted butter when you prepare it. Look for it in the freezer section of the supermarket with other prepared pastry and use it as a strudel wrap.

Grilling

Grill or broil, rather than fry, tender cuts of meat, chicken, and fish. Marinating first will add flavor, moisture, and tenderness. Grilling vegetables is a great way to bring out their flavor to the utmost.

Health food stores

Health food stores can be traps for the unwary. Check out the high-fat ingredients, such as hydrogenated vegetable oil, nuts, coconut, and palm kernel oil in products such as granola bars, fruit bars, and "healthy" cakes (even if made with whole-wheat flour) that they stock on their shelves.

Ice cream
A source of carbohydrate, calcium, riboflavin, retinol, and protein. Low-fat varieties have lower glycemic index values. Definitely a nutritious cold treat.

Jam
A tablespoon of jam on toast contains far fewer calories than a pat of butter. So, enjoy your jam and give fat the flick!

Keep jars of minced garlic, chili, or ginger in the refrigerator to spice up your cooking in an instant.

Lemon juice
Try a fresh squeeze with ground black pepper on vegetables instead of a pat of butter. Lemon juice provides acidity that slows gastric emptying and lowers GI values.

Milk
Many people dislike skim milk, particularly when they taste it on its own or in their coffee. However, you can use skim milk in a recipe and no one will notice—and the fat saving is great. For convenience you might want to keep powdered skim milk in the pantry; it can be made up to the desired quantity when you need it. It will taste more like fresh milk if you mix the powder and water according to directions and refrigerate the milk overnight before using it. Ultrapasteurized (or shelf-stable) milk is handy in the cupboard, too.

Nuts
Nuts are valuable for their vitamin E content, but they are also high in fat. To keep the fat content of a recipe low, the quantity of nuts has to be small.

Oil

Most of our recipes call for no more than two teaspoons of oil. Any polyunsaturated or monounsaturated oil is suitable. Cooking spray or brushing oil lightly over the base of the pan is ideal. If you find the amount of oil insufficient, cover your pan, or add a few drops of water and use steam to cook the ingredients without burning. It is a good idea to invest in a nonstick frying pan if you don't have one.

Pasta

A food to eat more of and a great source of carbohydrate and B vitamins. Fresh or dried, the preparation is easy. Just boil in water until tender or "al dente," drain, and top with a dollop of pesto, tomato sauce, or a sprinkle of Parmesan and pepper. There are many wonderful pasta cookbooks now available, and it's definitely worth investing in one to find all sorts of exciting ways to prepare this fabulous low-GI food. Pasta may appear in your menu as a side dish to meat, as noodles in soup, as a meal in itself with vegetables or sauce, or even as an ingredient in a dessert.

Questions

Ask your dietitian for more recipe ideas. (See page 130 in "For More Information" for guidance on finding a dietitian near you.)

Reduce the fat content of ground beef by browning it in a nonstick pan, then placing the meat in a colander and pouring boiling water through it to wash away the fat. Return to the pan to continue cooking. It is a good idea to buy the better-quality ground beef, which has less fat.

Stock
If you are prepared to go to the effort of making your own stock—good for you! Prepare it in advance, refrigerate it, then skim off the accumulated fat from the top. Prepared stock is available in long-life cartons and cans in the supermarket. Stock cubes are another alternative. Look for brands that have reduced salt.

To sauté
Heat the pan first, brush with the recommended amount of oil (or less), add the food and cook, stirring lightly over a gentle heat.

Underlying the need for fat is a need for taste. Be creative with other flavorings.

Vinegar
A vinaigrette dressing (1 tablespoon vinegar and 2 tablespoons of oil) with your salad can lower the blood-sugar response to the whole meal by up to 30 percent. The best types of vinegars for this purpose are red and white wine vinegar. You can also use lemon juice.

Weighing
What's the weight of the meat you're buying? Start noticing the weight that appears on the butcher's scales or package label and consider how many servings it will give you. With a food such as steak, which is basically all edible meat, 4 to 5 ounces per serving is sufficient. One pound is more than enough for four portions. Choose lean cuts of meat and trim away the fat before cooking or before you put it away. Alternate meat or chicken with fish once or twice a week.

Yogurt

Yogurt is a valuable food in many ways. It is a good source of calcium, "friendly bacteria," protein, and riboflavin, and, unlike milk, is suitable for people who are lactose intolerant. Low-fat plain yogurt is a suitable substitute for sour cream. If you're using yogurt in a hot sauce or casserole, add it at the last minute and do not let it boil, or it will curdle. It is best if you can bring the yogurt to room temperature before adding it to the hot dish. To do this, mix a small amount of yogurt with a little sauce from the dish, then stir this mixture back into the bulk of the sauce.

Zero fat

Eating zero fat is unhealthy, so speak with a dietitian about how to get just the amount you need. Our bodies need essential fatty acids that can't be synthesized and must be supplied in the diet. Fat does add flavor—use it to your advantage.

◀ 20 ▶

LET'S TALK GLYCEMIC LOAD

*I*N ADDITION TO the GI values we provide in this book, we also include the glycemic load (GL) value for average-sized food portions. Taken together, a food's GI value and glycemic load provide you with all the information you need to choose a diet brimming with health-boosting foods.

GLYCEMIC LOAD 101

A food's glycemic load results from the GI value and carbohydrate per serving of food. When we eat a carbohydrate-containing meal, our blood glucose first rises, then falls. The extent to which glucose rises and remains high is critically important to our health and depends on two things: the *amount* of a carbohydrate in the meal and the *nature* (glycemic index value) of that carbohydrate. Both factors equally determine blood-glucose changes.

Researchers at Harvard University came up with a way of combining and describing these two factors with the term "glycemic load," which not only provides a measure of the level of glucose in the blood, but also the insulin demand produced by a normal serving of the food. Researchers measure GI values for fixed portions of foods containing a certain amount of carbohydrate (usually 50 grams). Then, as people eat different-sized portions of the same foods, we can work out the extent to which a certain portion of food will raise the blood-glucose level by calculating a glycemic load value for that amount of food.

To calculate glycemic load, multiply a food's GI value by the amount of carbohydrate in a particular serving size, then divide by 100.

■

Glycemic load = (GI x carbohydrate per serving) ÷ 100

■

For example, a small apple has a GI value of 40 and contains 15 grams of carbohydrate. Its glycemic load is (40 × 15) ÷ 100 = 6. A small 5-ounce potato has a GI value of 90 and 15 grams of carbohydrate. It has a glycemic load of (90 × 15) ÷ 100 = 14. This means one small potato will raise your blood-glucose level higher than one apple.

Some nutritionists argue that the glycemic load is an improvement on the glycemic index because it provides an estimate of both quantity *and* quality of carbohydrate (the glycemic index gives us just quality) in a diet. In large Harvard studies, however, researchers were able to predict disease risk from people's overall diet, as well as its glycemic load. Using the glycemic load strengthened

How GI Values Affect Glycemic Load

THE GLYCEMIC LOAD is greatest for those foods that provide the highest-GI carbohydrate, particularly those we tend to eat in large quantities. Compare the glycemic load of the following foods to see how the serving size—as well as the GI value—helps to determine the glycemic response:

Rice, 1 cup
Carbohydrates: 43
GI: 83
GL: 36
$(83 \times 43) \div 100 = 36$

Spaghetti, 1 cup
Carbohydrates: 40
GI: 44
GL: 18
$(44 \times 40) \div 100 = 18$

the relationship, suggesting that the more frequently we consume high-carbohydrate, high-GI foods, the worse it is for our health. Carbohydrate by itself has no effect—in other words, there was no benefit to low carbohydrate intake over high carbohydrate intake, or vice versa.

■

Low GL = 10 or less
Intermediate GL = 11–19
High GL = 20 or more

■

If you make the mistake of using the GL alone, you might find yourself eating a diet with very little carbohydrate but a lot of fat and excessive amounts of protein. That's why you need to use the glycemic index to compare foods of similar nature (such as bread with bread) and use the glycemic load when you're deciding on the portion size of the carbohydrates you want to eat. If you use the technique correctly, GL values will guide you to eat smaller portions of high-GI foods.

Remember that the GL values we provide are for the standardized (nominal) portion sizes listed. If you eat a different portion size, then you'll need to calculate another GI value. Here's how: first, determine the size of your portion, then work out the available carbohydrate content of this weight (this value is listed next to the GL), then multiply by the food's GI value. For example, the nominal serving size listed for bran flakes is ½ cup, the available carbohydrate is 18 grams, and the glycemic index value is 74. So the GL for ½-cup serving of bran flakes is $(74 \times 18) \div 100 = 13$. If, however, you normally eat 1 cup of bran flakes, you'd need to double the available carbohydrate ($18 \times 2 = 36$) and the GL for your larger cereal portion would be $(74 \times 36) \div 100 = 27$. These numbers show that the larger portion of cereal releases a larger quantity of glucose into the bloodstream.

◀ 21 ▶

A TO Z GI VALUES

THE TABLE IN this section will help you find a food's glycemic index value quickly and easily, because we've listed the foods alphabetically.

The list provides not only the food's glycemic index value but also its glycemic load (GL = (carbohydrate content × GI) ÷ 100). We calculate the glycemic load using a nominal, or standardized, serving size as well as the carbohydrate content of that serving—both of which we've also listed. That way, you can choose foods with either a low GI value or a low glycemic load. If your favorite food is both high GI and high GL, you can either cut down the serving size or dilute the GL by combining it with very low-GI foods, such as rice and lentils.

For the first time, we've also included foods that have very little carbohydrate; their GI value is zero, indicated by [0]. Many vegetables, such as avocados and broccoli, and protein foods, such as chicken, cheese, and tuna, fall into the low- or no-carbohydrate category. Most alcoholic beverages are also low in carbohydrate.

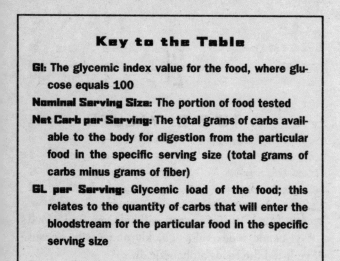

Key to the Table

GI: The glycemic index value for the food, where glucose equals 100

Nominal Serving Size: The portion of food tested

Net Carb per Serving: The total grams of carbs available to the body for digestion from the particular food in the specific serving size (total grams of carbs minus grams of fiber)

GL per Serving: Glycemic load of the food; this relates to the quantity of carbs that will enter the bloodstream for the particular food in the specific serving size

FOOD	GI Value	Nominal Serving Size	Net Carb per Serving	GL per Serving
A				
All-Bran®, breakfast cereal	30	½ cup	15	4
Almonds	[0]	1.75 oz	0	0
Angel food cake, 1 slice	67	¹⁄₁₂ cake	29	19
Apple, dried	29	9 rings	34	10
Apple, fresh, medium	38	4 oz	15	6
Apple juice, pure, unsweetened, reconstituted	40	8 oz	29	12
Apple muffin, small	44	3.5 oz	41	18
Apricots, canned in light syrup	64	4 halves	19	12
Apricots, dried	30	17 halves	27	8
Apricots, fresh, 3 medium	57	4 oz	9	5
Arborio, risotto rice, cooked	69	¾ cup	53	36
Artichokes (Jerusalem)	[0]	½ cup	0	0
Avocado	[0]	¼	0	0
B				
Bagel, white	72	½	35	25
Baked beans	38	⅔ cup	31	12
Baked beans, canned in tomato sauce	48	⅔ cup	15	7
Banana cake, 1 slice	47	⅛ cake	38	18
Banana, fresh, medium	52	4 oz	24	12
Barley, pearled, cooked	25	1 cup	42	11
Basmati rice, white, cooked	58	1 cup	38	22
Beef	[0]	4 oz	0	0
Beer	[0]	8 oz	10	0
Beets, canned	64	½ cup	7	5
Bengal gram dahl, chickpea	11	5 oz	36	4
Black bean soup	64	1 cup	27	17
Black beans, cooked	30	⅘ cup	23	7
Black-eyed peas, canned	42	⅔ cup	17	7

[0] indicates that the food has so little carbohydrate that the GI value cannot be tested. The GL, therefore, is 0.

FOOD	GI Value	Nominal Serving Size	Net Carb per Serving	GL per Serving
Blueberry muffin, small	59	3.5 oz	47	28
Bok choy, raw	[0]	1 cup	0	0
Bran Flakes™, breakfast cereal	74	½ cup	18	13
Bran muffin, small	60	3.5 oz	41	25
Brandy	[0]	1 oz	0	0
Brazil nuts	[0]	1.75 oz	0	0
Breton wheat crackers	67	6 crackers	14	10
Broad beans	79	½ cup	11	9
Broccoli, raw	[0]	1 cup	0	0
Broken rice, white, cooked	86	1 cup	43	37
Brown rice, cooked	50	1 cup	33	16
Buckwheat	54	¾ cup	30	16
Bulgur, cooked 20 min	48	¾ cup	26	12
Bun, hamburger	61	1.5 oz	22	13
Butter beans, canned	31	⅔ cup	20	6

C

FOOD	GI Value	Nominal Serving Size	Net Carb per Serving	GL per Serving
Cabbage, raw	[0]	1 cup	0	0
Cactus Nectar, Organic Agave, light, 90% fructose (Western Commerce)	11	1 Tbsp	8	1
Cactus Nectar, Organic Agave, light, 97% fructose (Western Commerce)	10	1 Tbsp	8	1
Cantaloupe, fresh	65	4 oz	6	4
Cappellini pasta, cooked	45	1½ cups	45	20
Carrot juice, fresh	43	8 oz	23	10
Carrots, peeled, cooked	49	½ cup	5	2
Carrots, raw	47	1 medium	6	3
Cashew nuts, salted	22	1.75 oz	13	3
Cauliflower, raw	[0]	¾ cup	0	0
Celery, raw	[0]	2 stalks	0	0
Cheese	[0]	4 oz	0	0

[0] indicates that the food has so little carbohydrate that the GI value cannot be tested. The GL, therefore, is 0.

FOOD	GI Value	Nominal Serving Size	Net Carb per Serving	GL per Serving
Cherries, fresh	22	18	12	3
Chicken nuggets, frozen	46	4 oz	16	7
Chickpeas, canned	42	⅔ cup	22	9
Chickpeas, dried, cooked	28	⅔ cup	30	8
Chocolate cake made from mix with chocolate frosting	38	4 oz	52	20
Chocolate milk, low-fat	34	8 oz	26	9
Chocolate mousse, 2% fat	31	½ cup	22	7
Chocolate powder, dissolved in water	55	8 oz	16	9
Chocolate pudding, made from powder and whole milk	47	½ cup	24	11
Choice DM™, nutritional support product, vanilla (Mead Johnson)	23	8 oz	24	6
Clif® bar (cookies & cream)	101	2.4 oz	34	34
Coca Cola®, soft drink	53	8 oz	26	14
Cocoa Puffs™, breakfast cereal	77	1 cup	26	20
Complete™, breakfast cereal	48	1 cup	21	10
Condensed milk, sweetened	61	2½ Tbsps	27	17
Converted rice, long-grain, cooked 20-30 min, Uncle Ben's®	50	1 cup	36	18
Converted rice, white, cooked 20-30 min, Uncle Ben's®	38	1 cup	36	14
Corn Flakes™, breakfast cereal	92	1 cup	26	24
Corn Flakes™, Honey Crunch, breakfast cereal	72	¾ cup	25	18
Corn pasta, gluten-free	78	1¼ cups	42	32
Corn Pops™, breakfast cereal	80	1 cup	26	21
Corn Thins, puffed corn cakes, gluten-free	87	1 oz	20	18
Corn, sweet, cooked	60	½ cup	18	11
Cornmeal, cooked 2 min	68	1 cup	13	9
Couscous, cooked 5 min	65	¾ cup	35	23

[0] indicates that the food has so little carbohydrate that the GI value cannot be tested. The GL, therefore, is 0.

FOOD	GI Value	Nominal Serving Size	Net Carb per Serving	GL per Serving
Cranberry juice cocktail	52	8 oz	31	16
Crispix™, breakfast cereal	87	1 cup	25	22
Croissant, medium	67	2 oz	26	17
Cucumber, raw	[0]	¾ cup	0	0
Cupcake, strawberry-iced, small	73	1.5 oz	26	19
Custard apple, raw, flesh only	54	4 oz	19	10
Custard, homemade	43	½ cup	26	11
Custard, prepared from powder with whole milk, instant	35	½ cup	26	9

D

FOOD	GI Value	Nominal Serving Size	Net Carb per Serving	GL per Serving
Dates, dried	50	7	40	20
Desiree potato, peeled, cooked	101	5 oz	17	17
Doughnut, cake type	76	1.75 oz	23	17

E

FOOD	GI Value	Nominal Serving Size	Net Carb per Serving	GL per Serving
Eggs, large	[0]	2	0	0
Enercal Plus™ (Wyeth-Ayerst)	61	8 oz	40	24
English Muffin™ bread (Natural Ovens)	77	1 oz	14	11
Ensure™, vanilla drink	48	8 oz	34	16
Ensure™ bar, chocolate fudge brownie	43	1.4 oz	20	8
Ensure Plus™, vanilla drink	40	8 oz	47	19
Ensure Pudding™, old-fashioned vanilla	36	4 oz	26	9

F

FOOD	GI Value	Nominal Serving Size	Net Carb per Serving	GL per Serving
Fanta®, orange soft drink	68	8 oz	34	23
Fettuccine, egg, cooked	32	1½ cups	46	15
Figs, dried	61	3	26	16
Fish	[0]	4 oz	0	0
Fish sticks	38	3.5 oz	19	7
Flan/crème caramel	65	½ cup	73	47
French baguette, white, plain	95	1 oz	15	15

[0] indicates that the food has so little carbohydrate that the GI value cannot be tested. The GL, therefore, is 0.

FOOD	GI Value	Nominal Serving Size	Net Carb per Serving	GL per Serving
French fries, frozen, reheated in microwave	75	30 pcs	29	22
French green beans, cooked	[0]	½ cup	0	0
French vanilla cake made from mix, with vanilla frosting	42	4 oz	58	24
French vanilla ice cream, premium, 16% fat	38	½ cup	14	5
Froot Loops™, breakfast cereal	69	1 cup	26	18
Frosted Flakes™, breakfast cereal	55	1 cup	26	15
Fructose, pure	19	1 Tbsp	10	2
Fruit cocktail, canned, light syrup	55	½ cup	16	9
Fruit leather	61	2 pcs	24	15
G				
Gatorade™ (orange) sports drink	89	8 oz	15	13
Gin	[0]	1 oz	0	0
Glucerna™, vanilla (Abbott)	31	8 oz	23	7
Glucose (dextrose)	99	1 Tbsp	10	10
Glucose tablets	102	3 pcs	15	15
Gluten-free corn pasta	78	1½ cups	42	32
Gluten-free multigrain bread	79	1 oz	13	10
Gluten-free rice and corn pasta	76	1½ cups	49	37
Gluten-free spaghetti, rice and split pea, canned in tomato sauce	68	8 oz	27	19
Gluten-free split pea and soy pasta shells	29	1½ cups	31	9
Gluten-free white bread, sliced	80	1 oz	15	12
Glutinous (sticky) rice, white, cooked	92	⅔ cup	48	44
Gnocchi	68	6 oz	48	33
Grapefruit, fresh, medium	25	1 half	11	3
Grapefruit juice, unsweetened	48	8 oz	20	9
Grape-Nuts® (Post), breakfast cereal	75	¼ cup	21	16

[0] indicates that the food has so little carbohydrate that the GI value cannot be tested. The GL, therefore, is 0.

FOOD	GI Value	Nominal Serving Size	Net Carb per Serving	GL per Serving
Grapes, black, fresh	59	¾ cup	18	11
Grapes, green, fresh	46	¾ cup	18	8
Green peas	48	⅓ cup	7	3
Green pea soup, canned	66	8 oz	41	27
H				
Hamburger bun	61	1.5 oz	22	13
Happiness™ (cinnamon, raisin, pecan bread) (Natural Ovens)	63	1 oz	14	9
Hazelnuts	[0]	1.75 oz	0	0
Healthy Choice™ Hearty 100% Whole Grain	62	1 oz	14	9
Healthy Choice™ Hearty 7-Grain	55	1 oz	14	8
Honey	55	1 Tbsp	18	10
Hot cereal, apple & cinnamon, dry (ConAgra)	37	1.2 oz	22	8
Hot cereal, unflavored, dry (ConAgra)	25	1.2 oz	19	5
Hunger Filler™, whole-grain bread (Natural Ovens)	59	1 oz	13	7
I				
Ice cream, low-fat, vanilla, "light"	50	½ cup	9	5
Ice cream, premium, French vanilla, 16% fat	38	½ cup	14	5
Ice cream, premium, "ultra chocolate," 15% fat	37	½ cup	14	5
Ice cream, regular fat	61	½ cup	20	12
Instant potato, mashed	97	¾ cup	20	17
Instant rice, white, cooked 6 min	87	¾ cup	42	36
Ironman PR® bar, chocolate	39	2.3 oz	26	10

[0] indicates that the food has so little carbohydrate that the GI value cannot be tested. The GL, therefore, is 0.

FOOD	GI Value	Nominal Serving Size	Net Carb per Serving	GL per Serving
J				
Jam, apricot fruit spread, reduced sugar	55	1½ Tbsps	13	7
Jam, strawberry	51	1½ Tbsps	20	10
Jasmine rice, white, cooked	109	1 cup	42	46
Jelly beans	78	10 large	28	22
K				
Kaiser roll	73	1 half	16	12
Kavli™ Norwegian crispbread	71	5 pcs	16	12
Kidney beans, canned	52	⅔ cup	17	9
Kidney beans, cooked	23	⅔ cup	25	6
Kiwi fruit	53	4 oz	12	7
Kudos® Whole Grain Bars, chocolate chip	62	1.8 oz	32	20
L				
Lactose, pure	46	1 Tbsp	10	5
Lamb	[0]	4 oz	0	0
Leafy vegetables (spinach, arugula, etc.), raw	[0]	1½ cups	0	0
L.E.A.N Fibergy™ bar, Harvest Oat	45	1.75 oz	29	13
L.E.A.N Life long Nutribar™, Chocolate Crunch	32	1.5 oz	19	6
L.E.A.N Life long Nutribar™, Peanut Crunch	30	1.5 oz	19	6
L.E.A.N Nutrimeal™, drink powder, Dutch Chocolate	26	8 oz	13	3
Lemonade, reconstituted	66	8 oz	20	13
Lentil soup, canned	44	9 oz	21	9
Lentils, brown, cooked	29	¾ cup	18	5
Lentils, green, cooked	30	¾ cup	17	5
Lentils, red, cooked	26	¾ cup	18	5

[0] indicates that the food has so little carbohydrate that the GI value cannot be tested. The GL, therefore, is 0.

FOOD	GI Value	Nominal Serving Size	Net Carb per Serving	GL per Serving
Lettuce	[0]	4 leaves	0	0
Life Savers®, peppermint candy	70	18 pcs	30	21
Light rye bread	68	1 oz	14	10
Lima beans, baby, frozen	32	¾ cup	30	10
Linguine pasta, thick, cooked	46	1½ cups	48	22
Linguine pasta, thin, cooked	52	1½ cups	45	23
Long-grain rice, cooked 10 min	61	1 cup	36	22
Lychees, canned in syrup, drained	79	4 oz	20	16
M				
M & M's®, peanut	33	15 pcs	17	6
Macadamia nuts	[0]	1.75 oz	0	0
Macaroni and cheese, made from mix	64	1 cup	51	32
Macaroni, cooked	47	1¼ cups	48	23
Maltose	105	1 Tbsp	10	11
Mango	51	4 oz	15	8
Maple syrup, pure Canadian	54	1 Tbsp	18	10
Marmalade, orange	48	1½ Tbsps	20	9
Mars Bar®	68	2 oz	40	27
Melba toast, Old London	70	6 pcs	23	16
METRx® bar (vanilla)	74	3.6 oz	50	37
Milk Arrowroot™ cookies	69	5	18	12
Millet, cooked	71	⅔ cup	36	25
Mini Wheats™, whole-wheat breakfast cereal	58	12 pcs	21	12
Mousse, butterscotch, 1.9% fat	36	1.75 oz	10	4
Mousse, chocolate, 2% fat	31	1.75 oz	11	3
Mousse, hazelnut, 2.4% fat	36	1.75 oz	10	4
Mousse, mango, 1.8% fat	33	1.75 oz	11	4
Mousse, mixed berry, 2.2% fat	36	1.75 oz	10	4
Mousse, strawberry, 2.3% fat	32	1.75 oz	10	3

[0] indicates that the food has so little carbohydrate that the GI value cannot be tested. The GL, therefore, is 0.

FOOD	GI Value	Nominal Serving Size	Net Carb per Serving	GL per Serving
Muesli bar containing dried fruit	61	1 oz	21	13
Muesli bread, made from mix in bread oven (ConAgra)	54	1 oz	12	7
Muesli, gluten-free, with low-fat milk	39	1 oz	19	7
Muesli, Swiss Formula	56	1 oz	16	9
Muesli, toasted	43	1 oz	17	7
Multi-Grain 9-Grain bread	43	1 oz	14	6
N				
Navy beans, canned	38	5 oz	31	12
Nesquik™, chocolate dissolved in low-fat milk, no-sugar-added	41	8 oz	11	5
Nesquik™, strawberry dissolved in low-fat milk, no-sugar-added	35	8 oz	12	4
New creamer potato, canned	65	5 oz	18	12
New creamer potato, unpeeled and cooked 20 min	78	5 oz	21	16
Noodles, instant "two-minute" (Maggi®)	46	1½ cups	40	19
Noodles, mung bean (Lungkow beanthread), dried, cooked	39	1½ cups	45	18
Noodles, rice, fresh, cooked	40	1½ cups	39	15
Nutella®, chocolate hazelnut spread	33	1 Tbsp	12	4
Nutrigrain™, breakfast cereal	66	1 cup	15	10
Nutty Natural™, whole-grain bread (Natural Ovens)	59	1 oz	12	7
O				
Oat bran, raw	55	2 Tbsp	5	3
Oatmeal, cooked 1 min	66	1 cup	26	17
Oatmeal cookies	55	4 small	21	12
Orange juice, unsweetened, reconstituted	53	8 oz	18	9

[0] indicates that the food has so little carbohydrate that the GI value cannot be tested. The GL, therefore, is 0.

FOOD	GI Value	Nominal Serving Size	Net Carb per Serving	GL per Serving
Orange, fresh, medium	42	4 oz	11	5
P				
Pancakes, buckwheat, gluten-free, made from mix	102	2 4" pancakes	22	22
Pancakes, made from mix	67	2 4" pancakes	58	39
Papaya, fresh	59	4 oz	8	5
Parsnips	97	½ cup	12	12
Pastry	59	2 oz	26	15
Pea soup, canned	66	8 oz	41	27
Peach, canned in heavy syrup	58	½ cup	26	15
Peach, canned in light syrup	52	½ cup	18	9
Peach, fresh, large	42	4 oz	11	5
Peanuts	14	1.75 oz	6	1
Pear halves, canned in natural juice	43	½ cup	13	5
Pear, fresh	38	4 oz	11	4
Peas, green, frozen, cooked	48	½ cup	7	3
Pecans	[0]	1.75 oz	0	0
Pepper, fresh, green or red	[0]	3 oz	0	0
Pineapple, fresh	66	4 oz	10	6
Pineapple juice, unsweetened	46	8 oz	34	15
Pinto beans, canned	45	⅔ cup	22	10
Pinto beans, dried, cooked	39	¾ cup	26	10
Pita bread, white	57	1 oz	17	10
Pizza, cheese	60	1 slice	27	16
Pizza, Super Supreme, pan (11.4% fat)	36	1 slice	24	9
Pizza, Super Supreme, thin and crispy (13.2% fat)	30	1 slice	22	7
Plums, fresh	39	2 medium	12	5
Pop Tarts™, double chocolate	70	1.8 oz pastry	36	25
Popcorn, plain, cooked in microwave oven	72	1½ cups	11	8

[0] indicates that the food has so little carbohydrate that the GI value cannot be tested. The GL, therefore, is 0.

POCKET GUIDE TO THE METABOLIC SYNDROME

FOOD	GI Value	Nominal Serving Size	Net Carb per Serving	GL per Serving
Pork	[0]	4 oz	0	0
Potato chips, plain, salted	54	2 oz	21	11
Potato, baked	85	5 oz	30	26
Potato, microwaved	82	5 oz	33	27
Pound cake (Sara Lee)	54	2 oz	28	15
PowerBar® (chocolate)	57	2.3 oz	42	24
Premium soda crackers	74	5 crackers	17	12
Pretzels	83	1 oz	20	16
Prunes, pitted	29	6	33	10
Pudding, instant, chocolate, made with whole milk	47	½ cup	24	11
Pudding, instant, vanilla, made with whole milk	40	½ cup	24	10
Puffed crispbread	81	1 oz	19	15
Puffed rice cakes, white	82	3 cakes	21	17
Puffed Wheat, breakfast cereal	80	2 cups	21	17
Pumpernickel rye kernel bread	41	1 oz	12	5
Pumpkin	75	3 oz	4	3
R				
Raisin Bran™, breakfast cereal	61	½ cup	19	12
Raisins	64	½ cup	44	28
Ravioli, meat-filled, cooked	39	6.5 oz	38	15
Red wine	[0]	3.5 oz	0	0
Red-skinned potato, peeled and microwaved on high for 6–7.5 min	79	5 oz	18	14
Red-skinned potato, peeled, boiled 35 min	88	5 oz	18	16
Red-skinned potato, peeled, mashed	91	5 oz	20	18
Resource Diabetic™, nutritional support product, vanilla (Novartis)	34	8 oz	23	8
Rice and corn pasta, gluten-free	76	1½ cups	49	37

[0] indicates that the food has so little carbohydrate that the GI value cannot be tested. The GL, therefore, is 0.

	GI Value	Nominal Serving Size	Net Carb per Serving	GL per Serving
Rice bran, extruded	19	1 oz	14	3
Rice cakes, white	82	3 cakes	21	17
Rice Krispies™, breakfast cereal	82	1¼ cups	26	22
Rice Krispies Treat™ bar	63	1 oz	24	15
Rice noodles, fresh, cooked	40	1½ cups	39	15
Rice, parboiled	72	1 cup	36	26
Rice pasta, brown, cooked 16 min	92	1½ cups	38	35
Rice vermicelli	58	1½ cups	39	22
Rolled oats	42	1 cup	21	9
Roll-Ups®, processed fruit snack	99	1 oz	25	24
Roman (cranberry) beans, fresh, cooked	46	¾ cup	18	8
Russet, baked potato	85	5 oz	30	26
Rutabaga, fresh, cooked	72	5 oz	10	7
Rye bread	58	1 oz	14	8
Ryvita® crackers	69	3 crackers	16	11

S

	GI Value	Nominal Serving Size	Net Carb per Serving	GL per Serving
Salami	[0]	4 oz	0	0
Salmon	[0]	4 oz	0	0
Sausages, fried	28	3.5 oz	3	1
Scones, plain	92	1 oz	9	8
Sebago potato, peeled, cooked	87	5 oz	17	14
Seeded rye bread	55	1 oz	13	7
Semolina, cooked (dry)	55	⅓ cup	50	28
Shellfish (shrimp, crab, lobster, etc.)	[0]	4 oz	0	0
Sherry	[0]	2 oz	0	0
Shortbread cookies	64	1 oz	16	10
Shredded Wheat™, breakfast cereal	75	⅔ cup	20	15
Shredded Wheat™ biscuits	62	1 oz	18	11
Skim milk	32	8 oz	13	4

[0] indicates that the food has so little carbohydrate that the GI value cannot be tested. The GL, therefore, is 0.

FOOD	GI Value	Nominal Serving Size	Net Carb per Serving	GL per Serving
Skittles®	70	45 pcs	45	32
Smacks™, breakfast cereal	71	¾ cup	23	11
Smoothie, raspberry (ConAgra)	33	8 oz	41	14
Snack bar, Apple Cinnamon (ConAgra)	40	1.75 oz	29	12
Snack bar, Peanut Butter & Choc-Chip (ConAgra)	37	1.75 oz	27	10
Snickers® bar	68	2.2 oz	35	23
Soda Crackers, Premium	74	5 crackers	17	12
Soft drink, Coca Cola®	53	8 oz	26	14
Soft drink, Fanta®, orange	68	8 oz	34	23
Sourdough rye	48	1 oz	12	6
Sourdough wheat	54	1 oz	14	8
Soy & Flaxseed bread (mix in bread oven) (ConAgra)	50	1 oz	10	5
Soybeans, canned	14	1 cup	6	1
Soybeans, dried, cooked	20	1 cup	6	1
Spaghetti, durum wheat, cooked 20 min	64	1½ cups	43	27
Spaghetti, gluten-free, rice and split pea, canned in tomato sauce	68	8 oz	27	19
Spaghetti, white, cooked 5 min	38	1½ cups	48	18
Spaghetti, whole wheat, cooked 5 min	32	1½ cups	44	14
Special K™, breakfast cereal	69	1 cup	21	14
Spirali pasta, durum wheat, al dente	43	1½ cups	44	19
Split pea and soy pasta shells, gluten-free	29	1½ cups	31	9
Split-pea soup	60	1 cup	27	16
Split peas, yellow, cooked 20 min	32	¾ cup	19	6
Sponge cake, plain	46	2 oz	36	17
Squash, raw	[0]	⅔ cup	0	0
Star pastina, white, cooked 5 min	38	1½ cups	48	18

[0] indicates that the food has so little carbohydrate that the GI value cannot be tested. The GL, therefore, is 0.

	GI Value	Nominal Serving Size	Net Carb per Serving	GL per Serving
Stay Trim™, whole-grain bread (Natural Ovens)	70	1 oz	15	10
Stoned Wheat Thins	67	14 crackers	17	12
Strawberries, fresh	40	4 oz	3	1
Strawberry jam	51	1½ Tbsps	20	10
Strawberry shortcake	42	2.2 oz	40	17
Stuffing, bread	74	1 oz	21	16
Sucrose	68	1 Tbsp	10	7
Super Supreme pizza, pan (11.4% fat)	36	1 slice	24	9
Super Supreme pizza, thin and crispy (13.2% fat)	30	1 slice	22	7
Sushi, salmon	48	3.5 oz	36	17
Sweet corn, whole kernel, canned, diet-pack, drained	46	1 cup	28	13
Sweet potato, cooked	44	5 oz	25	11
T				
Taco shells, baked	68	2 shells	12	8
Tapioca, cooked with milk	81	¾ cup	18	14
Tofu-based frozen dessert, chocolate with high-fructose (24%) corn syrup	115	1.75 oz	9	10
Tomato juice, canned, no added sugar	38	8 oz	9	4
Tomato soup	38	1 cup	17	6
Tortellini, cheese	50	6.5 oz	21	10
Tortilla chips, plain, salted	63	1.75 oz	26	17
Total™, breakfast cereal	76	¾ cup	22	17
Tuna	[0]	4 oz	0	0
Twix® Cookie Bar, caramel	44	2 cookies	39	17
U				
Ultra chocolate ice cream, premium, 15% fat	37	½ cup	14	5

[0] indicates that the food has so little carbohydrate that the GI value cannot be tested. The GL, therefore, is 0.

FOOD	GI Value	Nominal Serving Size	Net Carb per Serving	GL per Serving
Ultracal™ with fiber (Mead Johnson)	40	8 oz	29	12
V				
Vanilla cake made from mix, with vanilla frosting	42	4 oz	58	24
Vanilla pudding, instant, made with whole milk	40	½ cup	24	10
Vanilla wafers	77	6 cookies	18	14
Veal	[0]	4 oz	0	0
Vermicelli, white, cooked	35	1½ cups	44	16
W				
Waffles, Aunt Jemima®	76	1 4" waffle	13	10
Walnuts	[0]	1.75 oz	0	0
Water crackers	78	7 crackers	18	14
Watermelon, fresh	72	4 oz	6	4
Weet-Bix™, breakfast cereal	69	2 biscuits	17	12
Wheaties™, breakfast cereal	82	1 cup	21	17
Whiskey	[0]	1 oz	0	0
White bread	70	1 oz	14	10
White rice, instant, cooked 6 min	87	1 cup	42	36
White wine	[0]	3.5 oz	0	0
100% Whole Grain™ bread (Natural Ovens)	51	1 oz	13	7
Whole milk	31	8 oz	12	4
Whole-wheat bread	77	1 oz	12	9
Wonder™ white bread	80	1 oz	14	11
X				
Xylitol	8	1 Tbsp	10	1
Y				
Yam, peeled, cooked	37	5 oz	36	13

[0] indicates that the food has so little carbohydrate that the GI value cannot be tested. The GL, therefore, is 0.

	GI Value	Nominal Serving Size	Net Carb per Serving	GL per Serving
Yogurt, low-fat, wild strawberry	31	8 oz	34	11
Yogurt, low-fat, with fruit and artificial sweetener	14	8 oz	15	2
Yogurt, low-fat, with fruit and sugar	33	8 oz	35	12

[0] indicates that the food has so little carbohydrate that the GI value cannot be tested. The GL, therefore, is 0.

GLYCEMIC INDEX TESTING

$\mathcal{I}$F YOU ARE a food manufacturer, you may be interested in having the glycemic index value of some of your products tested on a fee-for-service basis. For more information, contact:

Sydney University Glycemic Index Research Service
(SUGiRS)
Department of Biochemistry
University of Sydney
NSW 2006 Australia
Fax: (61) (2) 9351-6022
E-mail: j.brandmiller@staff.usyd.edu.au

FOR MORE INFORMATION

To find a dietitian:
The American Dietetic Association
120 S. Riverside Plaza
Suite 2000
Chicago, IL 60606
Phone: 1-800-877-1600
www.eatright.org

**To order Natural Ovens bread
(available through mail-order only):**
Natural Ovens Bakery
PO Box 730
Manitowoc, WI 54221-0730
Phone: 1-800-772-0730
www.naturalovens.com

To order Fifty50 Foods:

Fifty50 Foods, Inc.
c/o Spectrum Foods, Inc.
PO Box 3493
Springfield, IL 62708
Phone: 1-800-238-8090
www.specialtyfoodpantries.com
www.fifty50.com

PRIMARY CARE PHYSICIANS

If you have heart disease or think you may have it, keep in close contact with your primary care physician or heart specialist.

WEIGHT LOSS ORGANIZATIONS

To help you lose weight, check the Yellow Pages under "Weight Control Services." Be aware, however, that not all weight-loss organizations are reputable. Check with your physician to make sure the group you'd like to join can help you lose weight safely.

HEART HELP

For more information about the prevention and treatment of stroke, heart disease, and related conditions, contact:

American Heart Association
7272 Greenville Avenue
Dallas, TX 75231
Phone: 1-800-AHA-USA1
http://www.americanheart.org

ACKNOWLEDGMENTS

W E WOULD LIKE to acknowledge the extraordinary efforts of Linda Rao, who adapted this book—and other books in The Glucose Revolution Pocket Guide series—for North American readers. She has worked to ensure that every piece of information is accurate and appropriate for readers in the U.S. and Canada.

ABOUT THE AUTHORS

JENNIE BRAND-MILLER, PH.D., is Professor of Human Nutrition in the Human Nutrition Unit, School of Molecular and Microbial Biosciences at the University of Sydney, and President of the Nutrition Society of Australia. She has taught postgraduate students of nutrition and dietetics at the University of Sydney for over twenty-four years and currently leads a team of twelve research scientists, whose interests focus on all aspects of carbohydrate—diet and diabetes, the glycemic index of foods, insulin resistance, lactose intolerance, and oligosaccharides in infant nutrition. She has published sixteen books and 140 journal articles and is the co-author of all books in the Glucose Revolution series.

■

KAYE FOSTER-POWELL, M. NUTR. & DIET., is an accredited practicing dietitian with extensive experience in diabetes

...nent. She has conducted research into the ,ycemic index of foods and its practical applications over the last fifteen years. Currently she is a dietitian with Wentworth Area Diabetes Services in New South Wales and consults on all aspects of the glycemic index. She is the co-author of all books in the Glucose Revolution series.

■

ANTHONY LEEDS, M.D., is Senior Lecturer in the Department of Nutrition & Dietetics at King's College London. He graduated in medicine from the Middlesex Hospital Medical School, London, in 1971. He conducts research on carbohydrate and dietary fiber in relation to heart disease, obesity, and diabetes, continues part-time medical practice, and is a member of the European Association of Scientific Editors. He chairs the research ethics committee of King's College London and in 1999 was elected a Fellow of the Institute of Biology. He is a co-author of the U.K. edition of *The Glucose Revolution*.

■

LINDA RAO, M.ED., a freelance writer and editor, has been writing and researching health topics for the past 16 years. Her work has appeared in several national publications, including *Prevention* and *USA Today*. She serves as a contributing editor for *Prevention* magazine and is the coadapter, with Johanna Burani, of all the titles in The Glucose Revolution Pocket Guide series. She lives in Allentown, Pennsylvania.